THE COMPLETE GOUT DIET AND NATURAL TREATMENT GUIDE

A 90 DAY PLAN TO LOWER URIC ACID,
ELIMINATE PAIN
AND LIVE GOUT FREE FOR LIFE

DAVID KELLER

The Complete Gout Diet and Natural Treatment Guide

Published by Feel Good Ink Books

First Edition

MEDICAL DISCLAIMER: This book is not intended as a substitute for medical advice from a qualified physician. The reader should regularly consult a physician in matters relating to their health, particularly with respect to any symptoms that may require diagnosis or medical attention. The author and publisher have made every effort to ensure accuracy of information but cannot be held liable for errors, omissions, or any consequences arising from the use of this information. Individual results may vary.

The stories in this book are composites based on real experiences, but names and identifying details have been changed to protect privacy.

CONTENTS

Introduction: Your Journey to Gout Freedom Starts Here ____ 4

Chapter 1: What They Don't Tell You About Gout ____ 12

Chapter 2: Your Body's Uric Acid Story ____ 22

Chapter 3: The 90-Day Framework ____ 38

Chapter 4: The First Seven Days ____ 52

Chapter 5: Week 2 - Building Momentum ____ 66

Chapter 6: Weeks 3-4 - Finding Your Rhythm & The Checkpoint ____ 80

Chapter 7: Weeks 5-8 - Expanding, Moving, and Navigating ____ 98

Chapter 8: Phase 2 Checkpoint & Trigger Testing ____ 120

Chapter 9: Weeks 9-10 - Personalizing Your Protocol ____ 140

Chapter 10: Weeks 11-12 - Advanced Optimization ____ 158

Chapter 11: Your Sustainable Maintenance Plan ____ 178

Chapter 12: The Complete 90-Day Review ____ 194

Appendix: Quick Reference Guides ____ 208

INTRODUCTION:

YOUR JOURNEY TO GOUT FREEDOM STARTS HERE

You're reading this book for one of two reasons: your toe is on fire right now, or you're terrified it will be again soon.

Maybe it's 3 AM and you literally can't bear the weight of your bedsheet. Maybe you just cancelled plans—again—because walking feels impossible. Maybe your doctor handed you a prescription, mumbled something about avoiding shrimp and beer, and sent you on your way.

Or maybe you're just exhausted. From the pain, the limitations, the constant anxiety about when the next attack will strike.

I get it. More importantly, the three people you're about to meet get it too.

Three People, One Breaking Point

Elena Martinez, 38, spent two years doing everything "right". She cut out red meat, seafood, and alcohol. She took her medication religiously. And she still hobbled through her daughter's soccer games, calling in sick to work, spending nights on the couch with ice packs while her 11-year-old made dinner.

Her breaking point came when her daughter Sofia asked, "Why are you always tired, Mom?"

Marcus Chen, 52, thought he could control his gout the same way he controlled everything else—with money and willpower. He hired nutritionists, bought expensive supplements, joined gyms. Nothing stuck.

His breaking point came at his daughter's wedding when he couldn't walk her down the aisle properly. Six months later, his son asked, "Dad, are you going to be around to meet your grandkids?"

James Morrison, 61, had resigned himself to gout. "This is just what happens when you get old," he told himself. He also had diabetes, kidney disease, and a previous heart attack. His doctors managed his symptoms but never explained why everything was connected.

His breaking point came when he couldn't get down on the floor to play with his grandson. "Why can't Grandpa play?"

Three different people. Three different breaking points. Same problem: they were treating symptoms instead of addressing the root cause.

Why This Book Is Different

This isn't a gout book. This is a metabolic health book that happens to fix your gout.

That distinction matters. Gout isn't really about uric acid crystals in your joints—that's just where the problem shows up. Gout is your body's alarm system screaming that something deeper is wrong with your metabolism.

Your insulin isn't working right. Your kidneys are struggling. Your inflammation is out of control. And your painful toe is just the most obvious symptom.

Fix the underlying metabolic dysfunction, and the gout takes care of itself.

What Happened to Elena, Marcus, and James

Let me jump to the ending first, because you deserve to know this works:

Elena is virtually pain-free after eleven months. She's lost 28 pounds without dieting, runs 5Ks with her daughter, and is actually present in her life again.

Marcus has been flare-free for six months, down 22 pounds. His diabetes is now controlled through diet alone—no medication. He's planning to cut back to a four-day work week because he finally understands that his health isn't negotiable.

James has lost 19 pounds. His kidney function has stabilized and actually improved for the first time in years. He's off diabetes medication and has been flare-free for seven months. He took his grandson fishing last month—the moment he thought he'd never have.

None of them are perfect. They all had setbacks. But 90 days later, they had their lives back.

The Four Pillars (And Why They Work Together)

Most gout advice fails because it treats these as separate issues. They're not. They're a system.

Pillar 1: Strategic Nutrition
Not "avoiding purines." Eating in a way that restores insulin sensitivity, reduces inflammation, and supports kidney function. You'll discover that some high-purine foods actually help, while some "safe" foods trigger attacks.

Pillar 2: Intelligent Hydration
Water is important, but it's not enough. You'll learn what to drink, when to drink it, and how to optimize your body's ability to flush uric acid efficiently.

Pillar 3: Movement That Heals
Exercise probably triggers your flares, so you stopped moving—which made everything worse. You'll learn the right movement at the right intensity that reduces inflammation and improves insulin sensitivity.

Pillar 4: Stress and Sleep Management
Stress raises cortisol, which raises uric acid. Poor sleep disrupts everything. You'll discover why every flare probably followed a stressful period, and what to do about it.

These four pillars address your metabolic dysfunction. Fix the metabolism, and the gout fixes itself.

The 90-Day Structure

This isn't a "change everything overnight" program. Your body didn't get here overnight, and it won't heal overnight either.

Phase 1: Foundation (Days 1-30)
Reset the basics. Clean up your diet, establish hydration habits, introduce gentle movement, start managing stress. This is where you'll see the quickest pain relief.

Phase 2: Integration (Days 31-60)
Expand your food variety, increase movement, test personal triggers, and integrate these habits into real life. Handle social situations, travel, and life's curveballs without derailing progress.

Phase 3: Mastery (Days 61-90)
Personalize the protocol to fit your life, optimize for maximum results, and build the sustainable system you'll use long-term. This is where the protocol becomes your lifestyle.

What to Expect (The Honest Version)

Week 1 will be hard. You'll be changing habits and probably feeling overwhelmed. You might question if this is worth it.

Week 2-3 will be better. Pain decreasing. Energy increasing. Sleep improving. You'll start believing this might work.

Week 4-6 might get frustrating. You'll hit a plateau or have a setback. This is where most people quit. You won't, because you'll know it's part of the process.

Week 7-9 will feel like breakthrough territory. Things click. You're not thinking about gout constantly anymore.

Week 10-12 will feel natural. You'll wonder why you didn't do this sooner.

Here's what I won't promise:

- That it's easy (it requires effort, especially at first)
- That it's fast (90 days might seem long, but lasting change takes time)
- That you'll never have another flare (life happens, but you'll have tools to manage it)

What I will promise: if you commit to this for 90 days—really commit—your pain will decrease, your health will improve, and your life will change.

How to Use This Book

Read the stories. Elena, Marcus, and James will show you what this journey really looks like—the struggles, wins, setbacks, and breakthroughs.

Follow the framework. Each chapter gives you the "what" and "why" before the "how." You'll understand the science so you're making informed decisions, not just following rules.

Take action. Every chapter ends with specific steps. Don't just read about change—make the change.

Be flexible. This isn't a rigid protocol. All three adapted this to fit their lives. You will too.

A Note About Your Doctor

This program is designed to work with your medical care, not replace it. You'll need your doctor for baseline labs, monitoring progress, and potentially adjusting medications as you improve.

Never stop or adjust medication without your doctor's guidance. As your metabolic health improves, you may need less medication. That's a conversation to have with your doctor.

Your 90-Day Commitment

Before you turn to Chapter 1, make a commitment—not to me, but to yourself:

I commit to giving this 90 days of genuine effort.

Not perfect effort. Just honest, consistent effort.

When it gets hard, I'll remember why I started.

When I have setbacks, I'll learn and adjust instead of quitting.

When I see results, I'll celebrate them and keep going.

90 days from now, I'll be someone who doesn't just manage gout—I'll be someone who's reclaimed my health and my life.

Elena was standing in her kitchen at 3 AM, exhausted and in pain, wondering if anything would ever change.

Marcus was watching his daughter's wedding video, seeing himself limp, feeling like a failure.

James was sitting at his grandson's birthday party, unable to play, accepting that this was just "old age."

They all stood at that crossroads. They all chose to try one more time.

90 days later, everything was different.

Your 90 days start now.

CHAPTER 1:

WHAT THEY DON'T TELL YOU ABOUT GOUT

Elena's Story: The Misdiagnosis Years

Elena Martinez stared at the prescription bottle in her hand. Allopurinol. Again.

This was the third doctor in two years to hand her the same medication, mumble something about avoiding red meat and beer, and shuffle out. The problem? She'd been taking allopurinol religiously for eighteen months. She didn't drink alcohol. And she'd already cut out red meat, seafood, and basically anything that once had a face.

Yet here she was at 3 AM on a Tuesday, her right big toe staging a full-scale rebellion.

"It's just gout," the first doctor had told her. "Take these pills, avoid purines, and you'll be fine."

But Elena wasn't fine. She was a 38-year-old single mother who could barely walk some mornings. She'd hobbled through her daughter's soccer games. She'd called in sick to work more times this year than in the previous five combined.

And the worst part? No one seemed to take her seriously.

"Maybe you're sneaking foods you shouldn't," her sister suggested.

"Are you sure you're not having beer on the weekends?" a colleague joked.

"Some people just have gout. It's genetic," her doctor shrugged.

That last statement was the only truthful thing anyone had told her. But it was also the most incomplete. Yes, genetics played a role. But saying "it's genetic" and walking away was like telling someone their house is on fire because they left the stove on, then leaving without mentioning they should probably turn it off.

The Truth They Should Have Told Her

Here's what Elena's doctors never explained: gout isn't really about eating too many shrimp or living like Henry VIII. Those things can trigger attacks, but they're not the root cause.

Gout is a metabolic disease

Not a dietary mistake. Not a character flaw. Not punishment for past sins.

Gout is your body's dramatic way of waving a red flag about deeper metabolic problems. When your car's check engine light comes on, the problem isn't the light bulb. The light is just the messenger. Gout is your body's check engine light, and that painful toe is trying to get your attention.

The Metabolic Cascade

Elena's body wasn't just producing too much uric acid. Her body was in metabolic chaos that had been building for years.

It started with insulin resistance. Elena didn't have diabetes—her blood sugar tests always came back "normal"—but her cells had slowly become resistant to insulin's signals. This forced her pancreas to pump out more and more insulin to do the same job.

Here's the part most doctors don't mention: **elevated insulin tells your kidneys to hold onto uric acid.** It's not malicious. It's just an unintended consequence of insulin's many jobs in the body.

So Elena's uric acid levels crept up. Year by year. Test by test. Until one day, her body reached its tipping point, and those uric acid crystals started forming in her joints.

But there's more to the story.

The 30 pounds Elena had gained over the past decade? That wasn't just about cookies. It was both a cause and consequence of the insulin resistance. The inflammation in her joints during gout attacks? That same inflammatory process was quietly damaging her blood vessels and organs between attacks.

Her occasional high blood pressure readings? Connected.

The fatty liver her doctor mentioned once and never brought up again? Connected.

The fact that she always felt tired, even after a full night's sleep? All connected.

This wasn't just gout. This was metabolic syndrome using her toe as the main stage.

Why This Matters to You

If you're reading this book, you're probably living some version of Elena's story. Maybe your gout is "under control" with medication, meaning you're taking pills every day and still getting attacks. Or maybe nothing seems to work long-term.

Here's the truth: **you cannot solve a metabolic disease with symptom management alone.**

Taking allopurinol without addressing the underlying metabolic dysfunction is like mopping the floor while the sink overflows. Sure, you're doing something. But the floor keeps getting wet.

This doesn't mean medication is bad. Elena still takes a lower dose today, and she's grateful it exists. But medication became dramatically more effective only after she addressed the root cause.

When she finally understood that gout was her body screaming about metabolic chaos, everything changed. Because metabolic problems have metabolic solutions.

The Four Pillars That Changed Everything

Two years after that 3 AM episode, Elena is virtually pain-free. She's been flare-free for eleven months. Her uric acid levels are healthy. She's lost 28 pounds without dieting. Her energy is back.

How? By addressing her metabolic health through four interconnected pillars:

Pillar 1: Strategic Nutrition Not "avoiding purines" but eating to restore insulin sensitivity, reduce inflammation, and support kidney function. Some high-purine foods actually helped, while some "safe" foods triggered attacks.

Pillar 2: Intelligent Hydration What she drank, when she drank it, and what she combined it with made the difference in how efficiently her kidneys eliminated uric acid.

Pillar 3: Movement That Heals The right type of movement, at the right intensity, actually reduced inflammation and improved insulin sensitivity. The key was knowing what "right" meant for her body.

Pillar 4: Stress and Sleep Management This was Elena's game-changer. When she discovered the cortisol-uric acid connection, her pattern of attacks suddenly made sense. Every flare had followed high stress and poor sleep.

These four pillars work together, not in isolation. That's what the next 90 days are about for you.

What Makes This Time Different

Elena had tried "lifestyle changes" before. She'd cut out foods. She'd tried to exercise. She'd bought a fancy water bottle.

But she'd tried them randomly, without understanding how they connected. She'd tried them alone, without support. And she'd tried them in addition to her already overwhelming life, not integrated into it.

This time will be different because:

You'll understand the why. Every change will make sense. You'll know how it addresses your metabolic dysfunction, not just your symptoms.

You'll have a system. Not a random collection of habits but a progressive, phased approach that builds on itself.

You'll have company. Throughout this book, you'll follow Elena's journey along with Marcus (a busy executive who thought he didn't have time for this) and James (a retiree managing multiple health conditions).

You'll start where you are. Elena didn't transform overnight. She started small. Some days were messy. She made mistakes. And she still succeeded.

The Medication Question

Let's talk about the pill bottle in your medicine cabinet.

Elena's doctors made allopurinol sound like the solution. Take this pill every day for life, and your gout will be "controlled." But they didn't tell her: allopurinol treats the symptom—elevated uric acid—not the cause.

Does that mean you should stop taking it? **Absolutely not.** Don't throw your medication away. Medication can be life-changing. Elena still takes it at a much lower dose.

But here's what changed: once she addressed the metabolic dysfunction, her medication became dramatically more effective. Her body was finally working with the medication instead of against it.

Think of it like trying to empty a bathtub with a cup while the faucet runs full blast. That's medication without metabolic healing. Turn off the faucet first, and suddenly the cup actually works.

Some people will be able to reduce or eliminate medication—always under medical supervision. Others will continue medication but at lower doses with better results. Some will stay on their current dose but finally get symptoms under control.

All three outcomes are wins. The goal isn't to be medication-free. The goal is to be pain-free and living the life you want.

What Elena Would Tell You Now

If you could sit down with Elena today over coffee, here's what she'd say:

"I wish someone had told me the truth from the beginning. Not to scare me, but to empower me. I wasted two years thinking my body was broken, when really it was trying to tell me something important.

"The first month was hard. I won't sugarcoat it. I had to relearn how to shop, how to cook. It was exhausting.

"I had moments where I wanted to give up. Where I stood in front of my fridge at 7 PM, tired from work, hungry, cranky, seriously considering just ordering pizza. For the record, I did order pizza twice. We're human.

"But somewhere around week three, something clicked. My pain decreased noticeably. My energy increased enough that I actually wanted to do things after work instead of collapsing on the couch. And I started to believe this could actually work.

"By day 60, I knew. This wasn't temporary. This was who I was becoming. And I liked this version of me better.

"By day 90, something even weirder happened: I wasn't following a protocol anymore. I was just living my life—a life that happened to include habits that kept me healthy. It stopped feeling like work and started feeling like just what I do.

"If I can do this while working full-time as a teacher, raising a daughter who thinks chicken nuggets are a food group, and living on a teacher's salary, you can do this too.

"The version of you that exists 90 days from now will thank you for starting today. I promise."

TAKE ACTION

Before moving to the next chapter, complete these three steps:

1. Complete Your Gout Profile Assessment (15 minutes)
Write down honest answers:

Your Current Reality:

- How many gout attacks in the past year?
- Worst pain level (1-10)?
- Current medications and dosages?
- How is gout affecting your daily life (work, family, hobbies, sleep)?

Your Health Context:

- Current weight and height?
- Other diagnosed conditions?
- Family history of gout?
- Stress level?
- Hours of quality sleep per night?

Your Why:

- What made you pick up this book today?
- What would be different in your life without gout attacks?
- What are you afraid will happen if you don't get this under control?
- What are you most looking forward to being able to do again?

2. Schedule Your Baseline Appointment

Call your doctor tomorrow and schedule an appointment for:

- Current uric acid level
- Comprehensive metabolic panel
- Lipid panel
- C-reactive protein (inflammation marker)

Tell your doctor you're starting a protocol to manage your gout and want baseline labs. Most doctors will support this.

3. Take Your Day 1 Measurements

Before you change anything, document where you are:

- Weight (same scale, same time of day)
- Take three photos: front, side, back
- Rate your current pain level (0-10)
- Rate your current energy level (0-10)
- Rate your current quality of life (0-10)

On day 90, you'll look back at these and be amazed.

Coming Up:

Chapter 2 introduces James—a 61-year-old retiree whose complex health history created the perfect storm for severe gout. His story will help you understand your lab results, the medication trap, and why addressing your metabolism works.

But before you turn the page, acknowledge something important: you just took the first step toward your gout-free future.

"The pain was the messenger, not the message. Once I understood what my body was really trying to tell me, everything changed." —Elena Martinez

---

CHAPTER 2:

YOUR BODY'S URIC ACID STORY

James's Story: The Perfect Storm

James Morrison was 49 years old when his heart stopped.

Not metaphorically. Actually stopped. In the middle of a Tuesday afternoon while he was running wire through an attic in July heat.

The heart attack wasn't massive, but it was real. Real enough to land him in the ICU. Real enough that Susan, his wife of 28 years, sat by his hospital bed and cried.

"You're going to retire early," she said. It wasn't a suggestion.

James survived. But the heart attack opened a Pandora's box of diagnoses. Once the doctors started looking, they found problems everywhere.

Type 2 diabetes. High blood pressure. High cholesterol. Fatty liver. And, almost as an afterthought, "elevated uric acid."

"Watch that," the cardiologist said, pointing at the lab result. "It can cause gout."

James had seven new prescriptions. He took them all dutifully. He changed nothing else. And he waited for the pills to fix him.

They didn't.

Three years later, at age 52, James woke up at 2 AM with his right big toe on fire. The pain was so intense he thought he'd broken it in his sleep.

Susan drove him to the emergency room. The doctor took one look, ordered a blood test, and said, "Looks like gout. Your uric acid is 9.8. That's high."

> James got another prescription. Allopurinol. Now he was taking eight medications daily.
>
> "This should control it," the doctor said.
>
> It didn't.

Twelve Years of Slow Decline

Over the next twelve years, James's health didn't improve. It got worse. Gradually, steadily, like a slow leak in a tire.

His weight crept up. 220 became 230 became 242.

His diabetes medications increased. Metformin wasn't enough. They added another.

His gout attacks became more frequent. Once a year became twice a year became three or four times a year.

His kidney function started declining. "Normal for your age and your diabetes," the doctor said. But the numbers kept going the wrong direction.

And through it all, he took his medications. Eight pills every morning. Four more at night. He did what he was told. He followed the rules.

But he kept getting worse.

At 61, retired for three years, James couldn't get down on the floor to play with his grandson without Susan helping him back up.

The moment that changed everything happened at Tyler's 5th birthday party.

Tyler asked, "Grandpa, will you play cars with me?"

James looked at the floor. The distance between standing and sitting seemed impossible. He knew if he got down there, he'd need help getting up. In front of everyone.

"Grandpa's too tired, buddy. Maybe later."

Tyler's face fell. Later never came.

That night, Susan found him in the garage, staring at nothing.

"I promised him I'd teach him to fish this summer," James said. "How am I supposed to do that when I can't even get in and out of a boat?"

"Then we fix this," Susan said. "Whatever it takes."

Understanding Your Lab Results

James had twelve years of lab results. Dozens of tests. Hundreds of numbers. But until he started looking at them differently, they were just numbers.

Let me show you what those numbers actually meant.

The Uric Acid Story

Uric acid is a waste product created when your body breaks down purines. Purines come from food and from your own cells dying and being replaced (which happens constantly).

Normally, your kidneys filter out uric acid and you pee it out. Problem solved.

But when your uric acid levels get too high—either because you're producing too much or your kidneys aren't eliminating enough—it crystallizes in your joints. Those crystals are sharp. Like tiny shards of glass. They trigger massive inflammation. That's a gout attack.

James's uric acid over time:

- Age 49 (heart attack): 8.1 mg/dL
- Age 52 (first gout attack): 9.8 mg/dL
- Age 55: 9.2 mg/dL (on allopurinol)
- Age 58: 10.1 mg/dL
- Age 61 (rock bottom): 10.1 mg/dL

Target range: Below 6.0 mg/dL (ideal), below 7.0 mg/dL (good)

James's uric acid was high at his heart attack. It got worse over twelve years despite medication. Why? Because medication treats the symptom without addressing why his body was producing so much and his kidneys weren't eliminating it efficiently.

The Kidney Function Story

Your kidneys filter about 50 gallons of blood daily, removing waste, balancing minerals, and regulating blood pressure. When they start failing, everything gets worse.

Two numbers tell your kidney function story:

Creatinine: Waste product that should be filtered out. Higher = worse kidney function.

eGFR (estimated Glomerular Filtration Rate): How well your kidneys filter blood. Lower = worse kidney function.

James's kidney function over time:

- Age 49: Creatinine 1.1, eGFR 72 (slightly below normal)
- Age 55: Creatinine 1.3, eGFR 58
- Age 58: Creatinine 1.4, eGFR 54 (Stage 3 kidney disease diagnosed)
- Age 61: Creatinine 1.4, eGFR 52

Normal eGFR: Above 90
Stage 3 kidney disease: 30-59 (James was here)
Stage 4: 15-29
Stage 5 (kidney failure): Below 15

James's kidneys were slowly failing. His doctor told him this was "expected progression" given his diabetes and gout. Nothing to be done except monitor and hope it stayed slow.

But here's what his doctor didn't emphasize: **failing kidneys make gout worse, and gout makes failing kidneys worse.** It's a vicious cycle.

Bad kidneys can't eliminate uric acid efficiently. High uric acid damages kidneys further. Round and round.

Breaking that cycle was key to James's recovery.

The Blood Sugar Story

Type 2 diabetes isn't really about blood sugar. That's just the symptom. It's about **insulin resistance.**

When you eat carbohydrates, your blood sugar rises. Your pancreas releases insulin. Insulin tells your cells to absorb that sugar and use it for energy.

But when your cells become resistant to insulin's signal (from years of too much sugar, too often), your pancreas has to release MORE insulin to do the same job. Eventually, your pancreas can't keep up. Blood sugar stays high. That's diabetes.

But here's the critical part: **high insulin tells your kidneys to hold onto uric acid.**

So James's diabetes wasn't just a separate condition. It was directly making his gout worse.

James's blood sugar over time:

- Age 49: Fasting glucose 168, A1C 8.2 (diabetes diagnosed)
- Age 55: Fasting glucose 158, A1C 8.0 (second medication added)
- Age 61: Fasting glucose 168, A1C 8.2 (right back where he started)

Normal ranges:

- Fasting glucose: 70-99 mg/dL
- A1C: Below 5.7%

Despite twelve years of increasing medication, James's blood sugar control got worse. The medications were managing symptoms but not fixing the underlying insulin resistance.

The Inflammation Story

Chronic, systemic inflammation damages everything. Your blood vessels, your organs, your joints. It's like a low-grade fire burning constantly throughout your body.

CRP (C-Reactive Protein): A marker of inflammation in your body.

James's inflammation:

- Age 49: CRP 8.2 mg/L
- Age 61: CRP 9.1 mg/L

Normal: Below 1.0 mg/L
Elevated: 1.0-3.0 mg/L
High: Above 3.0 mg/L

James's inflammation was through the roof. This wasn't just from gout attacks. This was systemic inflammation driving all his conditions: heart disease, diabetes, gout, kidney disease—all connected by inflammation.

Seeing the Connections

For twelve years, James saw his conditions as separate problems requiring separate medications:

- Heart disease → statin, aspirin
- Diabetes → metformin, another diabetes drug
- High blood pressure → lisinopril
- Gout → allopurinol, colchicine for flares
- Side effects → antacid

Eight medications. Zero addressing the root cause.

But his conditions weren't separate. They were all expressions of the same underlying problem: **metabolic dysfunction.**

Insulin resistance drove his diabetes. Insulin resistance told his kidneys to retain uric acid. High uric acid damaged his kidneys. Damaged kidneys couldn't eliminate uric acid. Chronic inflammation damaged his heart. Everything made everything worse.

It was all connected.

And that meant fixing one thing could help fix everything.

The Medication Trap

James isn't anti-medication. Medications saved his life after his heart attack. But he did fall into what he now calls "the medication trap": the belief that pills alone would fix his problems without him having to change anything.

How the Trap Works:

1. Get diagnosis (diabetes, gout, high blood pressure)
2. Get prescription
3. Take medication
4. Symptoms improve slightly (or don't)
5. Condition worsens over time
6. Get additional medication or increased dose
7. Repeat steps 4-6 indefinitely

James did this for twelve years. His medication list kept growing. His conditions kept worsening. And he kept thinking the next medication adjustment would finally fix everything.

What Medications Actually Do

Allopurinol: Reduces uric acid production by blocking the enzyme that creates it.

Does it work? Yes, for most people. James's uric acid did drop initially.

Does it fix gout? No. It manages one symptom without addressing why his body was producing so much or why his kidneys weren't eliminating it efficiently.

Metformin: Reduces glucose production in the liver and improves insulin sensitivity slightly.

Does it work? Yes, it lowers blood sugar.

Does it fix diabetes? No. It manages blood sugar without fixing the underlying insulin resistance. Which is why James needed more medication over time—the resistance kept worsening.

When Medications ARE Necessary

James wants to be clear: **Sometimes medications are necessary and life-saving.**

After his heart attack? He absolutely needed those medications. They kept him alive.

With Stage 3 kidney disease? He needed to protect his kidney function.

With severe gout attacks? Pain relief medication was essential.

The question isn't "medication or no medication." The question is: "Can I address the root cause so I need less medication, or can medications work better?"

For James, the answer was yes. But it required changing the things medications can't change.

Why Addressing Metabolism Works

Your body is constantly trying to maintain balance. When you cut yourself, your body heals it. When you get an infection, your immune system fights it. Your body has sophisticated systems for healing and maintaining itself.

But modern life overwhelms these systems: processed foods your body doesn't recognize, chronic stress, sedentary living, sleep deprivation, environmental toxins.

Your body is trying to heal. But you keep making it sick faster than it can heal.

The methods in this book aren't magic. They're removing obstacles to healing and providing what your body needs to do its job.

How Addressing Metabolism Helps Everything

Remember: James's conditions were all connected through metabolic dysfunction.

So fixing his metabolism helped everything:

Better insulin sensitivity →

- Blood sugar control improved
- Kidneys stopped retaining uric acid
- Inflammation decreased
- Weight came off
- Energy increased

Better kidney function →

- Uric acid elimination improved
- Blood pressure stabilized
- Waste products cleared efficiently

Reduced inflammation →

- Joint pain decreased
- Heart disease risk lowered
- Kidney protection
- Better sleep

One change created a cascade of improvements. This is what medications alone can't do—they target individual symptoms, not the underlying system.

What James Would Tell You Now

If you could sit down with James today—in his workshop, where he's building a birdhouse for Tyler—here's what he'd say:

"For twelve years, I waited for doctors and medications to fix me. They kept me alive, and I'm grateful for that. But they couldn't make me healthy. That was my job.

"I had to accept that my body didn't get here overnight, and it wasn't going to heal overnight. I'd spent decades eating wrong, moving wrong, stressing wrong, sleeping wrong. And medications couldn't undo decades of damage. Only time and consistent right choices could do that.

"I'm 61 years old. I have Stage 3 kidney disease. I had a heart attack twelve years ago. I'm not going to be a 25-year-old athlete. That's not the goal.

"The goal is: can I get down on the floor and play with my grandson? Can I teach him to fish? Can I work in my garden without needing a two-hour nap after? Can I do the things that make life worth living?

"The answer now is yes. Three months ago, it was no.

"My uric acid is down to 7.3. My kidney function improved—my doctor said that doesn't happen, but it did. My blood sugar is controlled with less medication. I've lost 19 pounds. I'm not in pain most days.

"But more than the numbers? I taught Tyler to fish last week. We caught two bass and he wouldn't stop talking about it.

"That's what this is about. Not perfect lab results. Living your life.

"If a 61-year-old retired electrician with a bad heart, bad kidneys, diabetes, and twelve years of gout can do this, you can too."

TAKE ACTION

Before moving to Chapter 3, complete these essential steps:

1. Gather Your Medical History

Collect your lab results from the past 12 months (or longer):

- Uric acid levels
- Kidney function (creatinine, eGFR)
- Blood sugar (fasting glucose, A1C if diabetic)
- Lipid panel (cholesterol, triglycerides)
- Inflammatory markers (CRP if available)
- Blood pressure readings

Create a simple tracking sheet:

Date	Uric Acid	Creatinine	eGFR	Fasting Glucose	A1C	BP	Weight

See the trend? Are things improving, stable, or worsening?

2. Complete Your Medication Inventory

List all current medications:

Medication Name	Dose	Frequency	What It's For	Side Effects

Also list:

- Over-the-counter medications you take regularly
- Supplements
- Herbal remedies

Important: Do NOT stop or change any medications without consulting your doctor. This inventory is for awareness and future discussion.

3. Identify Your Risk Factors

Check all that apply:

Medical conditions:

☐ Diabetes or pre-diabetes
☐ High blood pressure
☐ High cholesterol
☐ Kidney disease (any stage)
☐ Heart disease
☐ Fatty liver
☐ Obesity (BMI over 30)

Lifestyle factors:

☐ Sedentary lifestyle
☐ High-stress job or life situation
☐ Poor sleep (less than 6 hours or poor quality)
☐ Diet high in processed foods
☐ Regular alcohol consumption

The more boxes you checked, the more your conditions are interconnected. That's not bad news—it means fixing one thing can help everything.

4. Write Your Health Story

Take 10 minutes and write:

- When did this start?
- How has it progressed?
- What have you tried?
- What's your rock bottom moment?

- Why now? Why are you finally committed to change?
- What would your life look like without these health issues?

Keep this. You'll read it again on Day 90 and realize how far you've come.

Coming Up:

Chapter 3 gives you the complete framework for the next 90 days. You'll learn exactly how the four pillars work together, what to expect week by week, and why 90 days is the perfect timeline for transformation.

"My body was trying to tell me something for twelve years. I just wasn't listening. Once I started listening and responding, everything changed."
— James Morrison

CHAPTER 3:

THE 90-DAY FRAMEWORK

Marcus Discovers the System

Marcus Chen didn't believe in health coaches. He believed in data, systems, and results.

But Jennifer had made the appointment, and after six years of failed diet attempts, he'd agreed to go. Just once.

David's office didn't look like a typical wellness guru's space. No motivational posters. No incense. Just a whiteboard covered in diagrams and a desk stacked with research papers.

"Tell me what you've tried," David said.

Marcus pulled out his phone. "Keto for two months. Lost eight pounds, gained back twelve. Paleo for six weeks, couldn't sustain it. Whole30 twice—made it 23 days the first time, 17 the second. Hired a nutritionist last year who gave me meal plans I followed for three weeks before a business trip derailed everything."

"And?"

"And I'm still overweight. Still in pain. Still on four medications. Still limping at my daughter's wedding."

David nodded. "You sound like a high achiever."

"I am."

"And you're applying high-achiever thinking to health. Start hard, go perfect, push through, hit the goal, move on to the next project."

"That's how you succeed."

"All projects with endpoints. But health doesn't have an endpoint. You can't 'finish' being healthy. It's a system that runs continuously, not a project you complete."

Marcus leaned back. No wellness coach had ever told him he was thinking about this wrong.

"Let me show you something," David said, standing at the whiteboard. He drew four vertical lines. "These are pillars. Nutrition. Hydration. Movement. Stress Management."

"I've heard all this before."

"Have you? Or have you heard 'eat better and exercise more' and tried to willpower your way through it?"

Marcus stayed quiet.

"Here's what you've been missing: these aren't separate tasks. They're interconnected systems. Better nutrition improves sleep. Better sleep reduces stress. Less stress lowers cortisol. Lower cortisol helps your kidneys release uric acid. Everything affects everything."

David drew connections between the pillars. "When you improve one pillar, you make improving the others easier. When you ignore one, you sabotage the others. You can't out-diet your stress. You can't out-exercise your lack of sleep."

"So I need to do all four."

"Not perfectly. Consistently. There's a difference."

Marcus pulled out his laptop. "Show me the system."

For the next hour, David laid out the framework. Three phases. Ninety days. Progressive complexity. Built for real life, not controlled conditions.

By the time Marcus left, he had something he'd never had before: a roadmap he actually believed he could follow. Not because it was easy. Because it was systematic.

The Four Pillars: A System, Not a List

Most gout advice gives you lists. This is a system where everything works together.

Pillar 1: Strategic Nutrition

The Old Approach: Avoid purines. No red meat. No seafood. No alcohol. Follow this food list forever.

The Problem: You focus on what you CAN'T eat, feel deprived, eventually quit.

The New Approach: Eat to restore metabolic health. The right foods reduce inflammation, improve insulin sensitivity, and support kidney function. When your metabolism works, uric acid takes care of itself.

What this looks like:

Build every meal around this template:

Half your plate	Vegetables (especially greens and cruciferous)
Quarter plate	Quality protein (fish, poultry, eggs, occasional grass-fed meat)
Quarter plate	Healthy fats and complex carbs
Unlimited	Anti-inflammatory herbs, spices, lemon, olive oil

The foods that heal:

- Fatty fish (omega-3s fight inflammation)
- Berries and cherries (antioxidants reduce uric acid)
- Leafy greens (nutrients support kidney function)
- Cruciferous vegetables (aid liver detox)
- Quality proteins (maintain muscle, keep you full)
- Healthy fats (olive oil, avocados, nuts reduce inflammation)
- Beans and lentils (yes, despite purines—they're protective)

The foods that harm:

- Processed sugar (drives insulin resistance)
- Refined grains (spike blood sugar, worsen metabolism)
- Seed oils (vegetable, canola, soybean—highly inflammatory)
- Processed foods (additives trigger inflammation)
- Excessive alcohol, especially beer (directly raises uric acid)

Why this works: You're not just avoiding triggers. You're actively healing your metabolism.

Pillar 2: Intelligent Hydration

The Old Approach: "Drink more water."

The Problem: Water alone isn't enough. You need the right amount, with minerals, at the right times.

The Daily Protocol:

Morning (upon waking):

- 16 oz warm water with juice of half a lemon
- Add a pinch of sea salt (minerals matter)

Throughout the day:

- Aim for 80-100 oz total water
- Use three 32 oz bottles as visual tracking
- Bottle 1 done by noon, bottle 2 by 5 PM, bottle 3 by bedtime

Mid-morning and mid-afternoon:

- 8 oz unsweetened tart cherry juice

The mineral connection: Marcus drank 100 oz of water daily and felt terrible—exhausted, foggy, weak. Jennifer suggested adding a pinch of sea salt to his morning water. Within an hour, he felt better. The problem: he was diluting his electrolytes.

Get minerals from sea salt, leafy greens, avocados, nuts, and bone broth. Hydration isn't just about volume—it's about balance.

Pillar 3: Movement That Heals

The Old Approach: "Exercise more."

The Problem: Intense exercise can trigger gout flares. Lactic acid competes with uric acid for kidney elimination.

The New Approach: Gentle, consistent movement that improves metabolism without triggering attacks.

The Movement Principles:

Start where you are:

- James began with chair exercises
- Elena started with 10-minute walks
- Marcus began with hotel gym treadmill walking
- All three progressed from there

Consistency beats intensity:

- Daily 15-minute walk beats weekly 2-hour workout
- Gentle movement every day beats occasional intense bursts

Progress slowly:

- Increase by 10% per week maximum
- Pain the next day means you backed off too much
- Significant pain means you went too far

Why movement matters:

- Improves insulin sensitivity (directly lowers uric acid)
- Reduces systemic inflammation
- Supports kidney function
- Aids weight loss
- Reduces stress
- Promotes better sleep

The progression:

- **Phase 1:** Walking 10-15 minutes daily, gentle stretching
- **Phase 2:** Walking 15-25 minutes, adding variety, light strength work
- **Phase 3:** 20-30 minutes daily, sustainable activities you enjoy

Pillar 4: Stress and Sleep Management

Elena tracked everything—food, water, movement. Her logs were perfect. But she kept having unexplained pain spikes.

Until she started tracking stress.

Every spike followed high-stress periods. Parent-teacher conferences. Bills due. Sofia's friend drama. Work deadlines.

The connection: High stress → High cortisol → Kidneys retain uric acid → Pain increases

The Cortisol Problem:

Chronic cortisol:

- Tells kidneys to retain uric acid
- Increases systemic inflammation
- Disrupts sleep (which makes everything worse)
- Promotes insulin resistance

The Sleep Factor:
Poor sleep:

- Increases cortisol
- Spikes inflammation
- Reduces insulin sensitivity
- Impairs kidney function

James's kidney function improved when he started sleeping 7-8 hours consistently. His body finally had time to repair.

Practical Stress Management:
Find what works for YOU:

- **Elena:** 10-minute walks when stressed, evening work boundary
- **Marcus:** 5-minute morning meditation, no email after 9 PM
- **James:** Garden time, saying "no" to obligations

Sleep Basics:

- Same bedtime every night (even weekends)
- 7-8 hours minimum
- Dark, cool room (68°F or cooler)
- No screens 1 hour before bed

Marcus resisted this. He'd always "gotten by" on 5-6 hours. But when he started sleeping 7-8 hours, everything improved—energy, focus, pain, weight loss.

How the Pillars Work Together

Better nutrition → Stable blood sugar → Better sleep → Less stress → Easier to move

Better hydration → Efficient kidneys → Lower uric acid → More energy → Better exercise capacity

Better movement → Improved insulin sensitivity → Better blood sugar → Stress reduction → Deeper sleep

Better stress/sleep → Lower cortisol → Kidneys release uric acid → Better recovery → Easier to stick to nutrition

Everything affects everything. That's why half-measures don't work. But it also means improving one thing starts improving everything.

The Three-Phase Structure

Marcus wanted to know why three phases. Why not just do everything perfectly from day one?

Because that's how he'd failed every time before.

Phase 1: Foundation (Days 1-30)
Goal: Establish basic habits, see initial results, build belief

What you do:

- Remove inflammatory foods
- Establish hydration protocol
- Start gentle movement (10-15 minutes daily)
- Basic stress awareness

Expected by Day 30:

- 30-50% pain reduction
- 5-15 pounds lost (mostly water/inflammation)
- Energy noticeably better
- Sleep improving
- Belief that this actually works

The truth: Week 1 is hard. You're changing everything. But results come fast enough to keep you motivated.

Phase 2: Integration (Days 31-60)
Goal: Make this work in real life, not just controlled conditions

What you do:

- Expand food variety safely
- Master social situations (restaurants, parties, travel)
- Test personal triggers systematically
- Increase movement intensity

Expected by Day 60:

- Continued pain reduction (many pain-free by now)
- Additional 5-10 pounds lost
- Social confidence established
- Personal trigger knowledge
- Exercise routine feels natural

The truth: This is where you prove you can maintain this in the real world.

Phase 3: Mastery (Days 61-90)
Goal: Personalize everything, optimize, transition to lifestyle

What you do:

- Fine-tune all four pillars for YOUR body
- Personalize meal rotations
- Optimize exercise capacity
- Build sustainable maintenance

Expected by Day 90:

- Significant pain reduction or elimination
- Total weight loss 15-30+ pounds (varies widely)
- Lab markers dramatically improved
- Medication reductions (with doctor supervision)
- This feels completely natural

The truth: By Day 90, you're not finishing a program. You're just living your healthiest life.

Why 90 Days?

What happens over 90 days:

Days 1-21	Water weight drops, inflammation reduces, energy improves, habits feel like work
Days 22-45	Metabolic changes accelerate, insulin sensitivity improves, fat loss begins, habits feel more natural
Days 46-66	Significant metabolic shift, body composition changes, habits becoming automatic
Days 67-90	Metabolic health significantly improved, habits fully automatic, identity shift complete

Your body needs time to turn over cells, adapt metabolism, change gut bacteria, reduce chronic inflammation, and repair organ damage.

Your mind needs time to form lasting habits, change identity, build confidence, and master challenges.

90 days is long enough to work, short enough to commit to.

What Makes This Different

1. Addresses Root Cause, Not Symptoms

- **Others:** Avoid triggers, take medication, hope for best
- **This:** Fix the metabolic dysfunction causing high uric acid

2. Progressive, Not All-or-Nothing

- **Others:** Perfect from day 1, quit when you slip
- **This:** Build gradually, learn from setbacks, progress over perfection

3. All Four Pillars Together

- **Others:** "Just eat better" or "just exercise more"
- **This:** Nutrition, hydration, movement, and stress working as a system

4. Built for Real Life

- **Others:** Works in controlled settings, fails during stress
- **This:** Explicitly teaches restaurant navigation, travel, social situations

Your Commitment

Before you turn to Chapter 4, make a commitment—not to me, but to yourself:

I commit to giving this 90 days of genuine effort.

Not perfect effort. Just honest, consistent effort.

When it gets hard, I'll remember why I started. When I have setbacks, I'll learn and adjust instead of quitting. When I see results, I'll celebrate them and keep going.

90 days from now, I'll be someone who doesn't just manage gout—I'll be someone who's reclaimed my health and my life.

TAKE ACTION

Define Your Why
Not: "To lower my uric acid"

But: "So I can play with my grandchildren without pain. So I can travel with my wife. So I can live the second half of my life better than the first."

I'm committing to this because:

Set Your Start Date
Don't say "Monday" or "next month." Pick a specific date.

My Day 1 is: ______________________________

My milestones:

- Day 30: ______________________________
- Day 60: ______________________________
- Day 90: ______________________________

Identify Your Biggest Challenge
Be honest. What will be hardest?

My biggest challenge: ______________________________
My strategy: ______________________________

Build Your Team
Who's supporting you?

- Spouse/partner: ______________________________
- Accountability friend: ______________________________
- Doctor: ______________________________

Tell at least 3 people you're starting.

Coming Up:

Chapter 4 begins Phase 1. Where theory becomes action. Where planning becomes doing. You have your why. You have your framework. You have your commitment. Day 1 is coming.

"I've executed hundreds of business projects. This is just another project—except the product is my health, and the deadline is the rest of my life." — Marcus Chen

---

CHAPTER 4:

THE FIRST SEVEN DAYS

Day 1: The Beginning

Elena's Kitchen - Saturday Morning, 7 AM

Elena stood in her kitchen holding a trash bag, re-reading the pantry purge list for the third time. Sofia was still asleep, which was good because Elena was having a minor crisis.

The bag was supposed to be for donations. Instead, she found herself staring at a box of pasta like it had personally betrayed her.

"It's just pasta," she muttered. But it wasn't just pasta. It was the thing she made on Tuesday nights when she was too tired to think. It was the meal that took seven minutes and made her daughter happy.

And according to everything she'd learned, it was also spiking her blood sugar, driving her insulin up, and telling her kidneys to hold onto uric acid.

She put the pasta in the bag. Then took it out. Then put it back in.

Her phone buzzed. A text from the online support group: "Day 1 is the hardest. Just start. Don't aim for perfect."

She tied the bag and set it by the door before she could overthink it further.

Marcus's Kitchen - Saturday Morning, 6 AM

Marcus was already showered, caffeinated, and organized. He'd created a spreadsheet the night before with tabs for "Pantry Inventory," "Approved Foods," "Shopping List," and "Meal Prep Schedule."

His wife Jennifer walked into the kitchen, saw the spreadsheet open on his laptop next to a box of crackers, and laughed.

"You're making a project plan for cleaning out the pantry?"

"Efficiency," Marcus said. "If I'm doing this, I'm doing it right."

"You know this isn't a product launch, right? It's just food."

Marcus looked up. "My daughter's wedding was six weeks ago. I couldn't walk her down the aisle properly because my toe felt like it was on fire. This isn't 'just food.' This is me fixing a problem I should have fixed years ago."

Jennifer softened. "Okay. What do you need me to do?"

"Stop me from overthinking this."

She picked up the box of crackers and dropped it in the trash. "Like that?"

"That works."

James's Kitchen - Saturday Morning, 9 AM

James sat at the kitchen table while Susan moved through the pantry with surprising speed. She'd been ready for this.

"Do we really have to throw out the bread?" James asked.

"The white bread? Yes."

"What about the—"

"The sugary cereal? Also yes."

"Susan—"

"Jim, you sat at Tyler's birthday party and couldn't get on the floor with your grandson. You want to keep the cereal that's making you sick, or do you want to teach that boy to fish?"

James was quiet. "The fishing wins."

"Good answer." She softened her tone. "We're not throwing it all out. We're just making room for food that actually helps."

The Week 1 Framework: Foundation Reset

The first week isn't about perfection. It's about establishing three foundational habits:

1. **Removing inflammatory foods** that spike insulin and promote uric acid retention
2. **Adding anti-inflammatory foods** that support metabolic healing
3. **Establishing the hydration protocol** that helps your kidneys function optimally

That's it. Three things. Not thirty.

The Kitchen Overhaul (Days 1-2)

What Goes

The Primary Culprits:

- **Refined sugars and sweeteners** — Sodas, sweetened beverages, candy, cookies, anything with high fructose corn syrup
- **Refined grains** — White bread, white pasta, white rice, most crackers and chips
- **Processed seed oils** — Vegetable oil, canola oil, soybean oil (in almost every processed food)
- **Processed meats with additives** — Hot dogs, deli meats with nitrates, highly processed sausages

The Maybe Category:

- **Beer and alcohol** — All of it, for these 90 days
- **Fruit juices** — Replace with whole fruit
- **Low-fat and diet products** — They usually replace fat with sugar

What Stays (And What You Add)

Proteins:

- Eggs, chicken, turkey
- Fish (especially fatty fish like salmon, mackerel, sardines)
- Grass-fed beef in moderation
- Plain Greek yogurt

Fats:

- Olive oil, avocado oil, coconut oil
- Real butter (not margarine)
- Avocados
- Nuts and seeds

Vegetables:

- Everything green (leafy greens are unlimited)
- Cruciferous vegetables (broccoli, cauliflower, Brussels sprouts)
- Colorful vegetables (peppers, tomatoes, carrots)
- Root vegetables in moderation

Fruits:

- Berries (especially cherries and blueberries)
- Apples, pears, citrus fruits
- Limit to 2-3 servings daily

Other:

- Beans and lentils (despite being higher in purines, they're protective)
- Quinoa, wild rice, oats
- Coffee (good news!)
- Dark chocolate 70%+ (in moderation)

The Hydration Protocol (Days 3-7)

Water is necessary, but it's not sufficient. Your kidneys need specific support to eliminate uric acid efficiently.

The Daily Formula:

Morning (upon waking): 16 oz warm water with fresh lemon juice (half a lemon)

- Kickstarts kidney function
- Increases urine alkalinity which helps dissolve uric acid crystals

Throughout the Day: Minimum 80-100 oz of water, spread evenly

- Get a 32 oz water bottle
- Fill it three times
- First bottle done by noon, second by 5 PM, third by bedtime

Mid-Morning and Mid-Afternoon: 8 oz tart cherry juice (unsweetened)

- Anthocyanins reduce inflammation and may lower uric acid
- Timing matters—spread it out

Evening (optional): Herbal tea—ginger, nettle, or dandelion root

- All support kidney function
- Have anti-inflammatory properties

Days 3-7: Building Your Meal Rhythm

The Plate Formula:

Every meal should follow this basic structure:

- **Palm-sized portion of protein**
- **2-3 fists of vegetables**
- **Thumb-sized portion of healthy fat**
- **Optional: small serving of complex carbs**

Sample Week 1 Meals

Monday

Breakfast	3-egg omelet with spinach and mushrooms, half avocado, mixed berries
Lunch	Large salad with grilled chicken, olive oil/lemon dressing
Dinner	Baked salmon with roasted broccoli and quinoa

Tuesday

Breakfast	Greek yogurt with blueberries, walnuts, drizzle of honey
Lunch	Leftover salmon with side salad
Dinner	Chicken stir-fry with mixed vegetables over cauliflower rice

Wednesday

Breakfast	Smoothie (protein powder, frozen berries, spinach, almond butter, almond milk)
Lunch	Turkey and avocado lettuce wraps, carrot sticks
Dinner	Grass-fed burger patty (no bun) with sweet potato wedges and side salad

Thursday

Breakfast	Oatmeal with sliced apple, cinnamon, sliced almonds
Lunch	Leftover burger and vegetables
Dinner	Grilled chicken with Brussels sprouts and wild rice

Friday

Breakfast	2 eggs scrambled, sautéed spinach, half avocado, berries
Lunch	Large salad with leftover chicken
Dinner	Baked cod with asparagus and roasted bell peppers

Saturday

Breakfast	Veggie frittata (make extra for tomorrow), mixed berries
Lunch	Chicken vegetable soup (make a big batch)
Dinner	Sheet pan meal—chicken thighs with cherry tomatoes, zucchini, red onion

Sunday

Breakfast	Leftover frittata, avocado and berries
Lunch	Leftover soup with side salad
Dinner	Slow-cooked pot roast with carrots and celery, sautéed greens

Snacks (if needed):

- Apple with almond butter
- Handful of mixed nuts
- Vegetables with guacamole
- Hard-boiled eggs
- Greek yogurt with berries

What Went Wrong (And How to Fix It)

Elena's Day 5 Meltdown

By Thursday, Elena was exhausted. Sofia was complaining about the "weird" food. Meal prep was taking twice as long as expected. After work, staring at the chicken and vegetables she'd prepped, Elena seriously considered ordering pizza.

She didn't. But she also cried a little while cooking. Then she texted her support group: "This is so hard. Is it supposed to be this hard?"

The responses came immediately: "Week 1 is always the worst." "You're doing great." "It gets easier, I promise."

What helped: She stopped trying to make elaborate meals. Grilled chicken, steamed vegetables, done. Simple became her new standard.

The lesson: You don't have to be a chef. You just have to eat real food. Save the complicated recipes for when you have energy.

Marcus's Day 3 Near-Quit

Marcus almost quit on Tuesday. He'd scheduled a client dinner, forgot about it, and found himself at a steakhouse looking at a menu that might as well have been written in another language.

He ordered a steak (no sauce), steamed vegetables (no butter), and sparkling water. His client ordered wine and loaded mashed potatoes. The client seemed fine with it. Marcus felt awkward.

On the way home, he was furious at himself. For forgetting to plan. For feeling awkward. For caring what someone else thought about his food choices.

Then he checked his pain level. For the first time in months, it was a 2 instead of a 6.

He decided that was worth some awkwardness.

The lesson: Social situations will be weird at first. Your health is worth more than avoiding awkwardness.

James's Pleasant Surprise

James expected to be miserable. He expected to be hungry all the time. He expected to feel deprived and resentful.

By Day 7, he was... fine. Actually, better than fine.

His arthritis pain in his hands was noticeably better. He'd lost 4 pounds without trying. His blood sugar readings were the best they'd been in months. And he wasn't hungry because Susan was feeding him actual food with fat and protein instead of low-fat diet food that left him starving.

At church on Sunday, someone commented that he looked good. "What are you doing different?"

"Eating real food," he said. "That's it."

The lesson: Your body wants to heal. Sometimes you just need to stop getting in its way.

Week 1 Results: What to Expect

By the end of Week 1, here's what's realistic:

Pain/Inflammation:

- Slight to moderate decrease in baseline pain
- Joints may feel less "hot" or swollen
- Morning stiffness might improve
- Don't expect to be pain-free yet

Energy:

- First 2-3 days might feel rough (sugar withdrawal is real)
- Days 4-7 should show noticeable improvement
- Sleep quality often improves quickly

Weight:

- 2-5 pound loss is typical (mostly water weight from reduced inflammation)
- Don't obsess over the scale

Mood:

- Initial frustration and overwhelm (normal)
- By end of week: small sense of accomplishment
- Hope starting to return

Other Changes:

- Clearer thinking ("brain fog" lifting)
- Better digestion
- Reduced bloating
- More stable mood (less blood sugar crashes)

TAKE ACTION: Your Week 1 Checklist

Days 1-2: The Pantry Purge

☐ Remove refined sugars and sweeteners
☐ Remove refined grains
☐ Remove processed seed oils
☐ Remove alcohol
☐ Remove processed meats with additives

Day 3: Strategic Shopping

- ☐ Proteins: eggs, chicken, fish, grass-fed beef
- ☐ Vegetables (buy more than you think you need)
- ☐ Healthy fats: olive oil, avocados, nuts
- ☐ Tart cherry juice (unsweetened)
- ☐ Lemons (lots of them)

Days 3-7: Establish Your Rhythm

- ☐ Start every morning with lemon water
- ☐ Hit your hydration target daily (80-100 oz)
- ☐ Drink cherry juice mid-morning and mid-afternoon
- ☐ Follow the plate formula for every meal
- ☐ Prep extra at dinner for next day's lunch
- ☐ Track your pain levels daily (1-10 scale)
- ☐ Track your energy levels daily (1-10 scale)

Daily Tracking (Simple Version)

Date: ______________________________

Morning Pain Level (1-10): ______________________________

Evening Pain Level (1-10): ______________________________

Energy Level (1-10): ______________________________

Hydration Goal Met? (Y/N): ______________________________

Followed Meal Structure? (Y/N): ______________________________

Notes/Challenges: ______________________________

Coming Up:

Week 2 is where belief starts to replace scepticism. You'll build momentum, refine your hydration protocol, and start noticing changes others comment on.

Elena will discover batch cooking strategies that save her time and money. Marcus will successfully navigate his first business trip. James will start noticing changes in his arthritis pain that his doctor can't explain.

You've stuck with something for seven days. That's not nothing. That's everything.

"I expected Week 1 to be miserable. It was hard, but it wasn't miserable. By Day 7, I had hope for the first time in two years."

— Elena Martinez

CHAPTER 5:

WEEK 2 - BUILDING MOMENTUM

Day 10: Three Small Victories

Elena's Kitchen - Sunday Afternoon

"Mom, this is actually good."

Elena looked up from the cutting board where she was prepping vegetables. Sofia was eating leftover chicken stir-fry straight from the container.

"You said it was 'weird' three days ago."

"Yeah, but I was being dramatic. It's actually better than the old stuff." Sofia grabbed another forkful. "Are we doing the cooking thing again today?"

"We are. Want to help?"

Twenty minutes later, they had music playing, vegetables roasting, and chicken marinating. What surprised Elena most wasn't that the food was healthier—it was that this Sunday afternoon cooking routine with her daughter had become something they both looked forward to.

Two hours later: five containers of soup, three packages of grilled chicken, chopped vegetables for the week, a dozen hard-boiled eggs.

"That's it?" Sofia asked. "That's all we need?"

"That's most of our dinners and lunches. We just have to assemble them."

Sofia did the math. "So you're not stressed about dinner every night?"

"Exactly."

Marcus's Hotel Room - Monday Morning, Chicago

Marcus stood in his hotel room at 6 AM, looking at the mini fridge he'd requested. Inside: pre-cooked chicken, hard-boiled eggs, pre-cut vegetables, almonds, water bottles.

His assistant thought he was crazy. His wife helped him pack the cooler. The TSA agent gave him a strange look.

But now he had breakfast, lunch, and snacks. He wasn't at the mercy of conference room bagels.

His phone buzzed. Jennifer: *How's the food situation?*

Marcus: *I look ridiculous but it's working.*

Twenty minutes later, he was on a hotel treadmill. Just walking. Nothing intense. His toe didn't hurt. His energy was good. For the first time in years, he felt prepared instead of already exhausted.

James's Backyard - Sunday Morning

James stood in his backyard, looking at the raised garden bed he'd abandoned years ago when bending became too painful.

Susan came out with coffee. "What are you thinking?"

"I'm thinking I could plant a garden again."

"Your knees—"

"Are better. Not perfect, but better." He walked to the raised bed. "I can bend now. It hurts a little, but it's manageable."

Susan set down her coffee. "Jim, you've spent twelve years not doing things because you're afraid you'll have a flare. Maybe it's time to start doing things anyway."

That afternoon, they bought tomato starts, pepper plants, basil, and rosemary. He spent an hour working in the garden, moving slowly, taking breaks.

His knees were stiff afterward. His back was sore. But nothing was screaming.

He'd done something he loved. And his body had let him.

Refining Your Hydration

You've been doing the basic protocol for a week. Now we optimize it.

The Mineral Connection

Most gout advice says "avoid salt." But your body needs minerals to properly hydrate.

When you drink lots of water without adequate minerals, you dilute your electrolytes. This actually makes hydration less effective.

What you need:

- Sodium (yes, salt)
- Potassium
- Magnesium
- Calcium

Where to get them:

- Sea salt (pinch in morning lemon water)
- Leafy greens (potassium and magnesium)
- Avocados (potassium)
- Nuts and seeds (magnesium)

Marcus discovered this the hard way. Day 9, he felt exhausted despite drinking plenty of water. His wife suggested adding sea salt to his water. Within an hour, he felt better.

The issue wasn't dehydration. It was dilution.

Cherry Juice Timing

The basic protocol says cherry juice mid-morning and mid-afternoon. But adjust for your schedule:

- **If you work nights:** Adjust to your waking hours
- **If you have digestive issues:** Take it with food
- **If it's too sweet:** Dilute with water
- **If you can't find unsweetened:** Look for tart cherry concentrate

Elena found cherry juice on an empty stomach made her queasy. She started having it with her mid-morning snack. Problem solved.

Hydration Tracking That Works

Stop counting ounces. Use visual cues instead:

Get a 32 oz water bottle:

- Drink one before lunch (by noon)
- Drink one before dinner (by 5 PM)
- Drink one before bed (by 9 PM)

Three bottles = roughly 100 oz. Simple.

Check your urine color:

- Pale yellow = good
- Dark yellow = drink more
- Clear = might be overdoing it, add minerals

Movement Without Triggering Flares

Exercise triggers flares, so you stopped moving. But not moving makes everything worse.

The solution: the right movement at the right intensity.

Why Exercise Triggered Flares Before

Intense exercise creates lactic acid. Lactic acid competes with uric acid for kidney elimination. Uric acid backs up. Crystals form. Flare happens.

Also, exercising dehydrated or while eating inflammatory foods? Recipe for disaster.

But gentle, consistent movement in a metabolically healthier body? Doesn't trigger problems.

The 10-Minute Walking Protocol

Week 2 Goal: 10 minutes of walking daily
Not 30 minutes. Not an hour. Ten.

Best timing: After meals, especially dinner (helps blood sugar control)

Pace: Conversational. If you're breathing hard, slow down.

For Limited Mobility:

- Chair exercises (seated leg lifts, arm circles)
- Water exercise (pool walking)
- Gentle stretching

James started with chair exercises—five minutes twice daily. By Day 14, he was walking to the mailbox. By Day 20, around the block.

Progress is progress.

What Marcus Did Wrong

Day 12, Marcus felt great. He did 30 minutes on the elliptical at high intensity.

That night, his toe throbbed. Warning.

He backed off. Returned to 10-minute walks. By Day 18, he increased to 15 minutes. Slowly. Without problems.

The lesson: Feeling good doesn't mean invincible. Your body is healing, not healed.

The Social Navigation Guide: Part 1

Week 2 usually brings the first real social test.

Elena's Birthday Party Strategy

Sofia's 12th birthday party. Pizza and cake were non-negotiable.

Elena's plan:

- Eat a full meal before
- Have one slice of pizza (conscious choice)
- Skip cake or tiny piece
- Focus on watching Sofia, not eating

What happened:

- Ate before (success)
- One slice of pizza (success)
- Full piece of cake (not planned)
- Didn't beat herself up (biggest success)

Next day, she felt slightly off but no flare. Back on track immediately.

The lesson: One meal doesn't ruin everything. Getting back on track matters more than perfection.

Marcus's Client Dinner

Business dinner at a steakhouse. Three clients. Pressure to drink, to "enjoy himself."

Marcus's strategy:

- Reviewed menu online beforehand
- Decided on order in advance
- Had response ready for alcohol questions

What he ordered:

- Sparkling water with lime (looked like a cocktail)
- Ribeye steak, no sauce
- Steamed vegetables, side salad

When asked why he wasn't drinking: "Doc's got me on a medication thing. Can't mix it with alcohol."

Everyone laughed. No one pushed.

The lesson: Have a simple explanation ready. Most people don't actually care what you eat.

James's Church Potluck

Small town church potluck. Everyone notices everything.

James brought his own container of food. Grilled chicken, roasted vegetables, salad. Took small portions of "safe" dishes others brought.

Mrs. Henderson: "Jim, are you on one of those diets?"

"Doctor's orders. Trying to get my kidney numbers better."

"How's it going?"

"Actually working. Feeling better than I have in years."

Three other people wanted to know what he was doing. He'd shared his story with five people by lunch's end.

The lesson: People are more supportive than you expect. Your health improvement might inspire someone else.

Week 2 Challenges (The Real Talk)

The "Am I Doing This Right?" Anxiety

Around Day 10-12, most people second-guess everything.

Should I be drinking more water?
Is this protein amount too much?
Why did my friend lose 10 pounds and I only lost 3?

Stop. Breathe.

Your body isn't your friend's body. Your progress is your progress.

If you're eating real food, staying hydrated, moving daily, managing stress—you're doing it right.

The Scale Isn't Moving

Elena lost 6 pounds Week 1. Week 2? Zero.

She panicked. Almost gave up.

Then she noticed: belt notch down, jeans fitting better, face less puffy, ring looser.

Scale wasn't moving. Body was changing.

Remember: Weight is one metric. Not the most important one.

The Energy Dip

Days 10-12 often bring an energy dip. You felt great Days 7-9. Now you're tired.

This is normal. Your body is doing deep healing work. It's metabolically expensive.

Don't panic. Get more sleep. Keep going. By Day 14-15, energy usually returns.

Cravings Hit Hard

Day 11, Marcus wanted a beer desperately.

He called Jennifer. "I know I can't have it. I'm not going to. But I really want it."

"What do you actually want? The beer, or something else?"

He thought. "I want to relax. I want to feel normal."

"So go relax. Take a walk. Read. You don't need beer for that."

She was right. The craving passed in 20 minutes.

The lesson: Cravings often aren't about the food. They're about what you think it'll give you. Find another way.

Week 2 Results: What to Expect

By Day 14:

Pain/Inflammation:

- Continued reduction (6-7 range down to 3-4)
- Some days better than others (normal)
- Morning stiffness noticeably better

Energy:

- More stable throughout day
- Fewer crashes
- Mental clarity improving

Weight:

- Additional 2-4 pounds (total 5-10)
- Or no scale movement but body composition changing
- Clothes fitting better

Sleep:

- Falling asleep easier
- Staying asleep longer
- Waking refreshed

Mood:

- Less irritable
- More optimistic
- Believing this might work

TAKE ACTION: Your Week 2 Checklist

Daily Habits (Continue)

- Morning lemon water
- 80-100 oz hydration
- Cherry juice (adjusted timing)
- Plate formula meals
- 10 minutes walking

New This Week

- Add mineral support (sea salt in water)
- Batch cook one meal
- Navigate one social situation
- Try one new vegetable

Simple Tracking

Date: ___________

Pain AM/PM: ___ / ___

Energy: ___

Water Bottles: ___ / 3

Movement: ___ min

What Went Well: ____

What Was Hard: ____

Batch Cooking Essentials

Elena's Chicken Soup (6-8 servings)

- 2 lbs chicken
- 8 cups low-sodium broth
- 3 carrots, 3 celery stalks, 1 onion (chopped)
- 4 cloves garlic, 2 cups greens
- Thyme, salt, pepper

Simmer chicken in broth 20 min. Remove, shred. Add vegetables, simmer 15 min. Return chicken, add greens, cook 5 min.

Stores 5 days, freezes 3 months.

Marcus's Turkey Meatballs (20-24)

- 2 lbs ground turkey
- 1 egg, 1/2 cup almond flour
- 2 cloves garlic, Italian seasoning
- Salt, pepper

Mix, form balls, bake at 400°F for 20-25 minutes.

Stores 4-5 days, freezes 3 months.

Coming Up:

Week 3 is where you find your rhythm. Morning stretches, deeper stress management, and the shift from "I'm doing this" to "this is just who I am."

Elena will start a walking group. Marcus will discover meditation works. James will realize he's not constantly thinking about pain anymore.

You've made it two weeks. You've shown up consistently. You've proven you can do this.

Week 3 is where belief shifts from "I hope" to "this works."

"Week 2 was when I stopped white-knuckling it and started actually living it. The difference is everything." — Marcus Chen

---

CHAPTER 6:

WEEKS 3-4 - FINDING YOUR RHYTHM & THE CHECKPOINT

Day 17: Three Unexpected Moments

Elena's School - Wednesday Lunch Break

Elena was eating her packed lunch—leftover chicken and roasted vegetables—when Maria from the math department sat down.

"Okay, I have to ask. You look different."

Elena looked up. "Different how?"

"I don't know. Lighter? Happier? You've lost weight but it's more than that." Maria leaned in. "What are you doing?"

"Just eating better. Dealing with some health stuff."

"The gout thing?"

Elena was surprised Maria remembered. "Yeah. Turns out it's connected to a bunch of other things. Fixed the other things, gout's getting better."

"How much better?"

"I haven't had a flare in two weeks. I can walk without pain. I have energy again." Elena gestured at her lunch. "I'm eating real food, walking during lunch. That's basically it."

Three teachers were now listening.

"Wait," Carlos from history interrupted. "You're walking at lunch?"

"Yeah. Want to come tomorrow? Just 15 minutes. Nothing intense."

The next day, four teachers walked with her. By Friday, it was seven.

Elena wasn't trying to start anything. She was just walking. But apparently, her transformation was noticeable enough that others wanted in.

Marcus's Office - Thursday Morning

Marcus was in his office at 7 AM. Not unusual. What was unusual: he was sitting with his eyes closed, breathing deliberately.

Five minutes of meditation. That's all Jennifer had asked him to try. "Just five minutes before you start work."

He'd resisted. Meditation was for people with time. People who didn't have his responsibilities.

But he'd agreed to try for one week. Today was Day 4.

He set a timer. Sat. Closed his eyes. Focused on his breath.

His mind immediately flooded with his to-do list. The presentation. The email. The—

Breath in. Breath out.

His toe itched. This was stupid. He should be working.

Breath in. Breath out.

The timer went off. Five minutes done.

He opened his eyes and checked his body. Shoulders lower. Jaw unclenched. The frantic energy that usually drove his morning was... quieter.

He opened his email. Instead of feeling overwhelmed by 47 unread messages, he felt clear about which five actually mattered.

Okay. Maybe Jennifer was onto something.

James's Backyard - Saturday Morning

James was on his hands and knees in the garden, pulling weeds. His grandson Tyler was "helping" by digging holes in random places.

"Grandpa, what are we planting here?"

"Tomatoes. They'll be red when they're ready."

"Can I help water them?"

"Every day. That's your job."

Tyler beamed. Then, without warning, he tackled James in a hug. James, off balance, fell sideways onto the grass. Tyler landed on top of him, giggling.

A year ago, this would have been a disaster. The fall would have jarred his joints. He'd have been unable to get up without help.

But today, lying in the grass with his grandson laughing on top of him, James felt... fine. A little stiff when he stood up. Nothing more.

Susan was watching from the porch, wiping her eyes.

"What?" James called to her.

"You're playing. You're actually playing."

He looked down at Tyler, who was now making a mud pie. "Yeah. I guess I am."

The Stress-Pain Connection

You've been eating well for three weeks. You're hydrated. You're moving. So why did you wake up with more pain yesterday than you've had in a week?

Let me guess: you had a stressful day. A deadline. A fight. Bad news. Something that elevated your stress.

And the next day, your joints hurt.

This isn't coincidence. This is cortisol.

The Science (Simple Version)

Stressed = cortisol released. Cortisol is your "fight or flight" hormone. It's supposed to be temporary.

But modern life doesn't work that way. Traffic, deadlines, financial stress, relationship problems—your body interprets all of it as danger.

Chronic cortisol:

- Signals kidneys to retain uric acid
- Increases inflammation system-wide
- Disrupts sleep
- Promotes insulin resistance

You can eat perfectly and still trigger a flare if stress is out of control.

Elena's Stress-Eating Revelation

Day 19. Parent-teacher conferences all week. Sofia's friend drama. Bills due. Car made a weird noise.

Tuesday, Wednesday, Thursday—she ate well. Thursday night, she stood in front of the fridge at 9 PM and ate three spoonfuls of almond butter from the jar. Then leftover chicken. Then an apple. Then more almond butter.

She wasn't hungry. She was anxious.

Friday morning, her right toe was slightly swollen. Not a full flare, but a warning.

She texted her support group: "I didn't cheat with bad food. I just ate too much when stressed. Why does my toe hurt?"

Response: "Stress raises uric acid even without bad food. What's going on?"

That night, instead of eating when anxious, she walked. Just around the block. Ten minutes. When she came back, the anxiety had decreased enough that she could actually identify what she was feeling: overwhelmed, tired, worried.

She still had those problems. But she didn't make them worse by eating her feelings.

By Saturday, the swelling was gone.

The lesson: You can't out-eat your stress. But you can learn to recognize when stress is driving behavior instead of actual hunger.

Stress Management That Actually Works

Let's be honest: "stress management" sounds like another thing you don't have time for.

We're finding micro-strategies that fit into your actual life.

The 3-Minute Reset (Marcus's Discovery)

Marcus didn't have time for hour-long meditation. But he could do three minutes.

When stress spikes:

1. Stop what you're doing
2. Close your eyes
3. Take five slow, deep breaths (in for 4, out for 6)
4. Notice three things you can hear

5. Notice three things you can feel
6. Open your eyes

Three minutes. Doesn't solve your problems, but creates space between stress and reaction.

Marcus started doing this before big meetings. Before difficult conversations. It worked.

The Evening Boundary (Elena's Strategy)

Elena made one simple rule: no work after 8 PM.

She was a teacher. There was always more grading, planning, emails. She could work until midnight every night and still have more to do.

So she stopped trying. 8 PM, work closed. Even if it wasn't done.

First week was hard. She felt guilty. She worried she was falling behind.

Second week, she realized the work still got done. She was just more focused during work hours.

And her evenings? She spent them with Sofia. Reading. Watching shows. Just being present.

Her sleep improved. Her stress decreased. Her evening toe pain—the thing that had been showing up around 9 PM for months—disappeared.

The lesson: Boundaries aren't selfish. They're essential.

The Physical Release (James's Approach)

James found that stress lived in his body. Tight shoulders. Clenched jaw. Tension headaches.

He couldn't meditate. His mind was too busy. But he could move.

When stressed, he worked in his garden. The physical activity gave his stress somewhere to go.

If weather was bad, he did stretches. Simple ones. Just movement that reminded his body it wasn't in danger.

The lesson: Find what works for your personality. Not everyone de-stresses the same way.

Movement Progression (The Right Way)

You've been walking 10 minutes daily for two weeks. Your body has adapted. Time to progress.

But intelligently, not aggressively.

Week 3 Movement Goal: 15-20 Minutes Daily

Option 1: Extend your walk

- Keep same pace
- Just go a bit longer
- Still conversational intensity

Option 2: Add a second short session

- 10 minutes morning, 10 minutes evening
- Breaks up sitting time

Option 3: Add variety

- Walk 10 minutes
- Stretch 5-10 minutes

What Marcus Did Wrong (Again)

Day 20, Marcus felt great. He decided to test himself. Thirty minutes at higher intensity.

His knee hurt afterward. His toe was slightly swollen the next morning.

He'd pushed too hard, too fast. His cardiovascular system was ready. His joints weren't.

He backed off. Stayed at 15 minutes. Focused on consistency over intensity.

The lesson: Your cardiovascular fitness can improve faster than your joints can handle. Don't let your ego write checks your body can't cash.

Adding Stretching and Mobility Work

This is where James found his sweet spot. Walking was good, but stretching made the real difference for his stiffness.

Simple Morning Routine (5-10 minutes):

- Gentle neck rolls (both directions)
- Shoulder circles (forward and back)
- Arm crosses (gentle chest stretch)
- Seated toe touches (or as far as you can reach)
- Cat-cow stretches (if you can get on floor)
- Ankle circles (both directions)

Nothing intense. Nothing that causes pain. Just gentle movement that says "good morning" to your joints.

James did this every morning while his coffee brewed. By Week 3's end, his morning stiffness was almost gone.

The Comparison Trap

Day 18, James made the mistake of comparing himself to others in his online support group.

Someone posted: "Day 18, down 18 pounds!"

James had lost 8 pounds.

Someone else: "Completely pain-free for a week!"

James still had occasional stiffness.

Another: "Ran a 5K today!"

James was doing chair exercises.

He felt like a failure.

Susan found him staring at his phone, dejected. "What's wrong?"

"I'm not doing as well as everyone else."

"How old is the person who ran the 5K?"

"I don't know. Thirty-something?"

"Jim. You're 61. You have kidney disease, diabetes, and arthritis. You've had gout for twelve years. That thirty-something probably had gout for six months." She took his phone. "Stop comparing your Chapter 3 to someone else's Chapter 10."

She was right. His body had more healing to do. His progress was slower but it was still progress.

By Day 21, he'd lost another 2 pounds. His kidney function labs came back stable. His morning routine was feeling easier.

His progress. Not anyone else's.

The lesson: Your timeline is your timeline. Comparison steals joy. Focus on your own before-and-after.

Day 30: The First Checkpoint

Elena's Kitchen - Thursday Evening

Elena stood in her kitchen with two photos side by side on the counter.

Day 1: A woman who looked exhausted. Puffy face. Tired eyes. Shoulders slumped.

Day 30: A woman who looked alive. Clear face. Bright eyes. Standing tall.

Sofia walked in. "Are you looking at your pictures again?"

"Last time, I promise."

"You always say that." Sofia hugged her from behind. "But I get it. You look like a different person."

"I am a different person."

Elena pulled out her complete data log. Thirty days. Every meal. Every pain level. Every workout. Every struggle. Every victory.

Day 1 Stats:

- Weight: 178 lbs
- Pain: 8/10 average
- Energy: 3/10
- Sleep: 5 hours, poor quality

Day 30 Stats:

- Weight: 163 lbs
- Pain: 2/10 average
- Energy: 7/10
- Sleep: 7 hours, good quality

Fifteen pounds lost. But that wasn't the real story.

The real story: Yesterday, she chased Sofia around the park. Running. Laughing. Not thinking about pain. Just... being.

Two months ago, that was impossible. Today, it was normal.

Marcus's Doctor's Office - Thursday Afternoon

Dr. Patel stared at the lab results on his screen. Then at Marcus. Then back at the screen.

"These can't be right."

"What's wrong?"

"Nothing's wrong. That's the problem. These numbers are too good." He pulled up the comparison. "Your uric acid went from 9.2 to 7.1. Your fasting glucose from 142 to 108. Your triglycerides dropped 60 points."

Marcus felt his chest tighten. "What does that mean?"

"It means whatever you're doing, don't stop."

They discussed medication adjustments. Blood pressure medication reduced. Check back in 30 days to potentially reduce further.

Marcus walked out and sat in his car for ten minutes.

One month ago, he was limping at his daughter's wedding, on four medications, heading toward a heart attack like his father.

Today, he was reversing everything. Not managing. Reversing.

He called Jennifer. "The labs came back."

"And?"

"Dr. Patel says I'm reversing metabolic syndrome. He's reducing my medications."

He heard her crying on the other end.

James's Garden - Friday Evening

James stood in his garden holding a fishing rod. Tyler was beside him, practicing casting.

"Like this, Grandpa?"

"Exactly like that. Now flick your wrist—there! Perfect cast."

They were practicing for tomorrow's fishing trip. The real one. The one James had been promising for a year. The one he thought he'd never be physically able to do.

Susan watched from the porch, wiping her eyes.

Later, after Tyler left, James showed Susan his lab results.

Kidney function:

- One month ago: eGFR 52, Creatinine 1.4
- Today: eGFR 55, Creatinine 1.3

"Your kidneys improved," Susan said, staring at the numbers.

"The doctor said kidney function at my stage doesn't improve. He called me himself. Said he wanted to know exactly what I was doing."

James looked at his hands. "Sue, my hands don't hurt. I built that birdhouse for Tyler last week. I'm working in the garden for hours. I'm taking him fishing tomorrow and I'm not worried about whether I can do it. I know I can."

"How's your uric acid?"

"8.1. Not perfect, but down from 10.1. And I haven't had a flare in 28 days."

Susan hugged him. "You did it, Jim."

"We did it. You did this with me every step."

Your 30-Day Assessment

It's time to measure everything.

The Numbers

Weight and Measurements:

	Weight	Waist	Chest	Hips
Day 1				
Day 30				
Change				

Pain Tracking:

Day 1 Average: _____/10
Day 30 Average: _____/10
Pain-free days Week 1: _____
Pain-free days Week 4: _____

Energy Levels:

Day 1 Average: _____/10
Day 30 Average: _____/10

Sleep Quality:

Day 1: _____ hours, _____/10 quality
Day 30: _____ hours, _____/10 quality

Beyond the Numbers

Activities I couldn't do on Day 1 that I can do now:

1. ____
2. ____
3. ____

How I feel different (not just physically):

____

What others have said:

____

My proudest moment:

____

The Photo Comparison

Look at your Day 1 photos. Compare to Day 30.

What do you notice?

- Face less puffy? Y / N
- Better posture? Y / N
- Look healthier overall? Y / N
- More energy visible? Y / N

The photos don't lie. Neither do the measurements. But the real transformation is how you FEEL when you look at them.

What You've Learned

About Your Body

My biggest trigger foods: ______________________________

Foods I thought were bad but are fine: ______________________

My optimal sleep amount: ______________________________

How stress affects my pain: ____________________________

About Yourself

What surprised me most: ______________________________

What was easier than expected: __________________________

What was harder than expected: __________________________

How I've grown: ___________________________________

TAKE ACTION: Your 30-Day Checkpoint

Complete Assessment

- Take Day 30 photos (same poses as Day 1)
- Record all measurements
- Complete comparison worksheet
- Write your success story so far

Celebrate Appropriately

Choose a celebration that honors your journey:

- Buy new clothes that fit your transformed body
- Plan an activity you couldn't do on Day 1
- Share your story with someone who inspired you
- Do something physical that demonstrates your capability

Prepare for Phase 2

- Review what worked best in Phase 1
- Identify areas to focus on in Phase 2
- Schedule your Day 60 checkpoint date
- Commit to the next 30 days

Coming Up:

Phase 2 (Days 31-60) is about integration and expansion. You'll add food variety safely, navigate more complex social situations, and test your personal triggers systematically.

Elena will discover she can eat foods she thought were forbidden. Marcus will navigate international business travel. James will reduce medications for the first time in fifteen years.

You've completed Phase 1. You've reset the foundation. You've proven change is possible.

Now it's time to build on it.

"Day 30 was when I realized I wasn't doing this anymore. I WAS this. This was just who I am now." — Elena Martinez

"The numbers don't lie. My body is healing. At 52, I'm reversing damage I spent decades creating." — Marcus Chen

"My doctor said kidney function at my stage doesn't improve. But mine did. Never too late to heal." — James Morrison

---

CHAPTER 7:

WEEKS 5-8 - EXPANDING, MOVING, AND NAVIGATING

Day 31: Three New Beginnings

Elena's Kitchen - Saturday Morning

"Mom, are we eating chicken again?"

Elena looked up from her meal prep. Sofia wasn't complaining, just observing. They'd had chicken four times this week.

"You're right. I've been playing it safe." Elena pulled out her phone and scrolled through the recipe folder she'd been saving. "What if we tried something new this week?"

"Like what?"

"How about lamb? Or duck? Or—wait, here's a lentil curry recipe."

"Lentils have purines though, right? I thought those were bad."

Elena had thought so too. But her research revealed something interesting: plant-based purines don't affect uric acid the same way animal purines do. In fact, legumes might actually be protective.

"Want to be my taste tester?"

By Sunday evening, they'd made three new recipes: a lentil curry, salmon with a different preparation, and roasted vegetables with spices Elena had never used.

Sofia's verdict: "The curry is weird but good. Can we make that again?"

Elena realized she'd been so focused on "not messing up" that she'd stopped being creative. Phase 1 was about establishing safety. Phase 2 was about expansion.

Time to expand.

Marcus's Home Office - Sunday Evening

Marcus was researching restaurants in Austin. He had a conference next week—three days, multiple client dinners, hotel food.

Phase 1, he'd brought all his own food and felt ridiculous. Phase 2, he needed a more sustainable approach.

Jennifer walked in. "Still planning?"

"I can't bring a cooler on every business trip for the rest of my life."

"So don't. You know what to order now. You know what works."

He pulled up the restaurant menu. Steakhouse. He could do this.

- Steak (no sauce, or sauce on side)
- Grilled vegetables
- Side salad with olive oil
- Sparkling water

Same strategy as before, but this time he wasn't panicking. He was planning.

The difference? Five weeks of data. Five weeks of success. Five weeks of proof that he could do this.

"I think I'm ready," he said.

"I know you are."

James's Garden - Sunday Afternoon

James stood in his garden surveying his work. The tomatoes were starting to flower. The peppers had small buds. Everything was growing.

Susan came out with iced tea. "Looking good."

"You know what I realized? I've been eating the same seven meals for five weeks."

"They're working though."

"They have. But I'm bored." He sipped the tea. "What if we tried some different fish? Or maybe that quinoa thing you mentioned?"

"Who are you and what have you done with my husband?"

James laughed. "I'm just saying, if this is how I'm eating for the rest of my life, I should probably learn to enjoy it more."

That evening, Susan made lentil soup with vegetables from their garden. James was skeptical—lentils were on every "avoid" list he'd seen.

But his body didn't react. No pain. No swelling. Just a full stomach and a satisfied sense that maybe the rules weren't as rigid as he'd thought.

The Truth About Food Variety

Phase 1: you ate the same safe foods repeatedly because you were terrified of triggering a flare.

Chicken. Salmon. Broccoli. Salad. Repeat.

It works. But it's not sustainable long-term. Eventually, you get bored. Eventually, you crave variety. Eventually, the restriction feels like deprivation.

Phase 2 solves this by teaching you to expand intelligently.

The Purine Paradox

Everything you've read says "avoid high-purine foods." But the research tells a more nuanced story.

Animal purines vs. Plant purines:

Foods like organ meats, certain fish, and game meats contain purines that DO increase uric acid and trigger flares.

But foods like lentils, beans, mushrooms, spinach, and asparagus also contain purines—yet multiple studies show they DON'T increase gout risk. Some actually decrease it.

Why? The fiber, antioxidants, and other compounds in plant foods counteract the purine content.

What this means:

- Organ meats, sardines, anchovies: still avoid
- Lentils, beans, mushrooms, spinach: actually safe (and beneficial)

Elena discovered this when she tried lentil curry. No reaction. James found the same with lentil soup. Both had been avoiding legumes unnecessarily.

Protein Rotation

You've probably been eating chicken and salmon on repeat. Time to expand.

Safe proteins to add:

Poultry:

- Duck (yes, it's fatty, that's fine)
- Turkey breast, thighs, ground
- Cornish hen

Seafood:

- Cod, halibut, tilapia (white fish)
- Shrimp in moderation (many people tolerate it fine)
- Scallops, crab, lobster

Red Meat (grass-fed, moderate portions):

- Lamb (surprisingly well-tolerated)
- Bison (leaner alternative)
- Continue beef in moderation

The key: Quality matters more than type. Grass-fed, wild-caught, organic when possible.

The Seafood Exception

Traditional gout advice says avoid all shellfish. But research shows this is oversimplified.

Marcus discovered he could eat shrimp without problems. James found scallops worked well. Elena had no issues with crab.

The way to know? Test systematically (covered later).

Expanding Vegetables and Fruits

Vegetables You Might Have Been Avoiding:

Mushrooms: High in purines, but multiple studies show no increased gout risk. Rich in vitamin D.

Asparagus: Same story. High in purines, but actually protective.

Spinach: Despite purine content, associated with LOWER gout risk in studies.

Add these:

- Purple cabbage (anthocyanins)
- Rainbow chard
- Beets (anti-inflammatory)

- Artichokes
- Bok choy

The more colorful your plate, the more antioxidants you're getting.

Fruits: The Sweet Spot

You've been limiting fruit to 2-3 servings daily. That's still the guideline, but expand variety.

Add:

- Kiwi (vitamin C supports uric acid excretion)
- Papaya (anti-inflammatory enzymes)
- Pineapple (bromelain reduces inflammation)
- Watermelon (hydrating, alkalizing)
- Citrus variety

Flavor Without Inflammation

Phase 1 was about removing inflammatory foods. Phase 2 is about adding flavor through anti-inflammatory ingredients.

The Spice Cabinet Expansion

Beyond the basics (turmeric, ginger, garlic, cinnamon), add:

- **Cumin:** Anti-inflammatory, aids digestion
- **Coriander:** Helps blood sugar regulation
- **Cardamom:** Anti-inflammatory, adds sweetness
- **Fennel:** Aids digestion, slightly sweet
- **Sumac:** Tangy, lemony, high in antioxidants

Marcus discovered that well-seasoned food didn't need sauces. A properly spiced chicken breast was better than one drowned in teriyaki sauce.

Umami Without MSG

Natural umami boosters:

- Mushrooms (especially dried shiitake)
- Tomato paste
- Miso paste (fermented, probiotic benefits)
- Coconut aminos (soy sauce alternative)
- Nutritional yeast (B vitamins, cheesy flavor)

These add depth and satisfaction without inflammatory additives.

Weeks 5-6: The Expansion Protocol

Week 5: Add One New Protein, Three New Vegetables

New protein options:

- Try duck, lamb, or a fish you haven't had
- Test shrimp or scallops if you've been avoiding them

New vegetables:

- Add mushrooms if you've been avoiding them
- Try asparagus
- Add a purple or dark-colored vegetable

Method:

- Add ONE new food at a time
- Wait 24-48 hours to assess response
- Track any changes in pain, energy, digestion
- If no negative response, add to rotation

Elena tried lamb for the first time in Week 5. She was nervous—red meat had always been on the "avoid" list. But she chose grass-fed lamb chops, grilled them with rosemary, and waited.

No flare. No pain increase. Just a delicious dinner that wasn't chicken.

Week 6: Add New Flavors and Cooking Methods

New cooking methods:

- If you've been grilling everything, try roasting
- Try slow-cooking (set it and forget it)
- Try sheet-pan meals (minimal cleanup)

New flavor profiles:

- Try an Indian curry
- Make Mexican with cumin, coriander, lime
- Try Mediterranean with za'atar and lemon
- Experiment with Asian flavors (ginger, garlic, coconut aminos)

James discovered that slow-cooking made even tough cuts tender. Marcus found that sheet-pan meals took 10 minutes of prep. Elena learned that curry could be as simple as coconut milk, curry powder, and whatever protein and vegetables she had.

Variety doesn't have to be complicated.

Fine-Tuning Your Exercise Routine

Day 47: Elena's Breakthrough

Elena stood at the staff meeting feeling restless. Not anxious restless. Energy restless.

The principal was droning on about testing protocols. Elena's mind wandered to the 5K registration form she'd bookmarked.

Six weeks ago, she could barely walk 10 minutes. Now she was walking 25 minutes daily, and yesterday she'd jogged—actually jogged—for 30 seconds just to see if she could.

No pain. No swelling. Just her, moving faster than a walk, feeling like she was flying.

At lunch, she mentioned it to the walking group. "I'm thinking about signing up for the Cherry Blossom 5K in April."

"I'll do it with you," Maria said immediately.

By the end of lunch, seven teachers had committed. Elena had accidentally started a running club.

That afternoon, she downloaded a Couch to 5K app. But not the regular version. She'd modify it. Go slower. Listen to her body. Not push too hard.

She had twelve weeks until race day. Plenty of time to build up safely.

Marcus's Hotel Gym - Thursday Morning, Denver

Marcus set the treadmill to 3.5 mph and a 3% incline. Six weeks ago, this would have been his maximum. Now it was his warm-up.

He'd been in Denver for three days. His hotel gym routine was now as automatic as brushing his teeth.

5:30 AM: gym opens. 5:35 AM: Marcus on treadmill.

Fifteen minutes walking (warm-up). Ten minutes strength training (bodyweight exercises he'd learned from YouTube). Five minutes stretching. Done by 6 AM. Shower, breakfast, ready for the day.

The revelation wasn't that he could exercise while traveling. It was that exercise made travel easier. Better energy. Less jet lag. Clearer thinking. Stress management built into his morning.

He increased the treadmill to 4.0 mph. Then 4.5 mph. He was jogging. Lightly, but jogging.

His toe didn't hurt. His knee felt fine. His breathing was controlled.

After five minutes, he brought it back down to 3.5 for recovery, then back up to 4.0 for another five minutes.

Interval training. Gentle intervals, but still.

He finished feeling energized, not exhausted. That was the key: exercise should give energy, not deplete it.

James's Backyard - Thursday Afternoon

James was digging a new garden bed. Had been for an hour. His back was tired but not screaming. His hands were sore but functional. His knees were holding up.

This would have been impossible two months ago.

Susan came out with water. "You've been out here all afternoon."

"I know. Feels good."

The garden work had become James's primary exercise. Digging, weeding, hauling soil, bending, stretching. Functional movement that served a purpose beyond "working out."

He'd also added morning stretches while his coffee brewed. Ten minutes of gentle movement to wake up his joints.

Chair exercises in winter. Walking in spring and fall. Garden work in summer. James had found his year-round movement routine, and none of it felt like "exercise." It felt like living.

Understanding Exercise and Gout

Why Exercise Triggered Flares Before

When you exercise intensely:

- Lactic acid production increases
- Lactic acid competes with uric acid for kidney elimination
- Uric acid backs up temporarily
- Crystals form, flare happens

Also: intense exercise is a stressor. Cortisol rises. Cortisol tells kidneys to retain uric acid.

Put it together: intense exercise + dehydration + metabolic stress + poor underlying health = flare.

But: **gentle, consistent exercise in a body that's metabolically healthier doesn't trigger these problems.**

Why Movement Helps Now

You've spent 6+ weeks improving your metabolic health. Your insulin sensitivity is better. Your inflammation is lower. Your kidneys function more efficiently.

Movement improves insulin sensitivity. Every time your muscles contract, they become more sensitive to insulin.

Movement reduces systemic inflammation. Regular gentle exercise is anti-inflammatory.

Movement supports weight loss. Less weight means less joint stress.

The key is finding the intensity that helps without hurting.

The Exercise-Inflammation Sweet Spot

Think of exercise intensity on a spectrum:

Too Little (Sedentary):

- Insulin resistance worsens
- Muscle loss accelerates
- Joint stiffness increases
- Gout risk increases

Just Right (Goldilocks Zone):

- Improves insulin sensitivity
- Maintains/builds muscle
- Reduces inflammation
- Decreases gout risk

Too Much (Overtraining):

- Produces excess lactic acid
- Increases cortisol chronically
- Increases inflammation
- Can trigger gout flares

Signs You're in the Zone:

- Energy increases after exercise
- Slight muscle soreness next day (not pain)
- Sleep improves
- Mood improves
- No joint swelling or increased pain
- Looking forward to next session

Signs You're Pushing Too Hard:

- Exhausted for hours after

- Significant joint pain
- Swelling in affected joints
- Sleep disrupted
- Dreading next session

Marcus learned this the hard way. Week 6, he felt great and pushed to 30 minutes of hard treadmill work. His toe swelled that evening. He'd crossed from "just right" into "too much."

He backed off, rebuilt slowly, and found his personal threshold: 30 minutes total, with no more than 10-15 minutes at elevated intensity, always with recovery periods.

Progressive Overload: The 10% Rule

You can't do the same workout forever. Your body adapts. You need progressive overload—gradually increasing the challenge.

But with gout, progress conservatively.

The 10% Rule: Increase your total weekly exercise volume by no more than 10% per week.

Week 7: 20 minutes daily = 140 minutes weekly
Week 8: Add 10% = 154 minutes weekly (22 minutes daily)

This feels slow. That's the point. Slow progress is sustainable progress.

What to increase:
Option 1: Duration (same intensity, just longer)

Option 2: Frequency (same duration, more often)

Option 3: Intensity (gentle hills, short jogging intervals)

Pick ONE variable at a time. Don't increase duration AND intensity simultaneously.

Elena increased duration first. Marcus increased intensity first. James increased frequency. All three progressed differently. All three avoided setbacks.

Navigating Social Situations

Week 5-8 usually brings more complex social challenges.

Elena's First Date - Friday Evening

Elena stood in front of her closet, trying to decide what to wear. First date in three years. She was nervous, but not about the usual first-date things.

She was nervous about the restaurant.

David had suggested Italian. Elena had researched the menu online, identified three safe options, and practiced her order in her head. But what if he ordered wine? What if he suggested sharing appetizers?

Sofia appeared in the doorway. "You look stressed."

"I'm not stressed."

"You're doing that thing with your hands."

"Okay, maybe a little stressed."

"Is it because of your food thing?"

"It's not a 'food thing.' I'm just eating healthy."

"So tell him that. If he's weird about it, he's not the right guy anyway." Sofia shrugged. "That's what you always tell me about friends."

When did her eleven-year-old become so wise?

An hour later, Elena sat across from David (different David, not the health coach) at the Italian restaurant.

"The carbonara here is supposed to be amazing," David said. "Want to split it?"

Here it was. The first test.

"It looks great, but I'm actually going to get the grilled salmon. I've been eating really clean lately and feeling so much better."

"Oh yeah? What prompted that?"

"Health stuff. I had some issues with inflammation and changed how I eat. Made a huge difference."

"That's cool. My sister did something similar for her autoimmune thing. The salmon looks good. I might get that too."

And just like that, it was fine. No judgment. No weird questions. Just... normal.

At the end of the night, he walked her to her car. "I had a great time. Want to do this again?"

"Yes," Elena said. And she meant it.

Driving home, she realized: she'd spent weeks dreading social situations, convinced everyone would judge her food choices. But most people were too worried about their own stuff to care about hers.

The fear had been worse than the reality.

Marcus's Business Trip Success

Austin. Three days. Five client meals.

Day 1 - Steakhouse:

- Ordered: Ribeye (no sauce), grilled asparagus, side salad (olive oil and vinegar)
- Drank: Sparkling water with lime
- Result: Perfectly satisfied, no issues

Day 2 - Italian:

- Ordered: Grilled branzino, sautéed spinach, roasted vegetables
- Skipped: Bread, pasta, dessert
- Result: Clients ordered pasta, he enjoyed his fish, no one cared

Day 3 - Mexican:

- Ordered: Fajitas (no tortillas), extra vegetables and guacamole, side of black beans
- Made: Basically a burrito bowl
- Result: Delicious, filling, no problems

The key? He stopped apologizing or explaining. He just ordered what worked for him. No one questioned it.

James's Church Potluck Reality

Small town church potluck. Everyone knows everyone.

James brought his own container of food. Grilled chicken, roasted vegetables, salad. He took small portions of a few "safe" dishes others brought.

Mrs. Henderson asked, "Jim, are you on one of those diets?"

"Doctor's orders. Trying to get my kidney numbers better."

"Oh honey, good for you. How's it going?"

"Actually working. Feeling better than I have in years."

Three other people at church wanted to know what he was doing. By the end of lunch, he'd shared his story with five people.

The lesson: People are more supportive than you expect. And your health improvement might inspire someone else.

Restaurant Mastery by Cuisine

Let's get tactical. Here's exactly how to order at different restaurants.

The Universal Restaurant Strategy

Before you go:

1. Look up menu online
2. Identify 2-3 safe options
3. Have backup plan

When you order:

1. Be clear and confident
2. Request substitutions without apologizing
3. Ask for sauce on side
4. Don't over-explain

Key phrases:

- "Could I substitute [vegetable] for [potato/rice/pasta]?"
- "Could I get that with sauce on the side?"
- "I'll have [protein] with extra vegetables, please."

Quick Guide by Cuisine

Mexican: Fajitas (no tortillas, extra vegetables), carne asada, burrito bowl (skip rice, no cheese, extra guac)

Italian: Grilled fish/chicken, cioppino, caprese salad, grilled vegetables (skip bread and pasta)

Asian: Stir-fries (sauce on side), steamed fish, Thai curry (light rice), lettuce wraps

Steakhouse: Steak, grilled chicken, salmon, salads, steamed vegetables (skip bread and loaded potatoes)

Indian: Tandoori proteins, chicken tikka, vegetable curry, dal (skip or limit naan and rice)

Mediterranean: Everything works—grilled fish, lamb, chicken souvlaki, Greek salad, vegetables

Weeks 5-8 Sample Meal Plans

Week 5: Protein Expansion

Monday	Pan-seared duck breast (new!) with roasted root vegetables
Tuesday	Lamb chops (new!) with rosemary, asparagus, sweet potato
Wednesday	Shrimp stir-fry (testing shellfish) with mixed vegetables
Thursday	Bison burgers (new!) with roasted Brussels sprouts
Friday	Cod with lemon-herb butter, roasted asparagus
Saturday	Slow-cooker pot roast with carrots, parsnips
Sunday	Sheet-pan chicken with purple cabbage, peppers

Week 6: Flavor Expansion

Monday	Coconut curry chicken (new flavor!) with cauliflower rice
Tuesday	Mexican-spiced beef with peppers, black beans, guac
Wednesday	Miso-glazed salmon with bok choy
Thursday	Za'atar chicken with roasted Mediterranean vegetables
Friday	Slow-cooker Thai curry with chicken and vegetables
Saturday	Grilled lamb kebabs with tzatziki, cucumber salad
Sunday	Sheet-pan sausage with Brussels sprouts, butternut squash

TAKE ACTION: Weeks 5-8 Checklist

Food Expansion

- ☐ Test one new protein per week
- ☐ Try three new vegetables
- ☐ Experiment with new spices/flavors
- ☐ Try one new cooking method

Movement Progression

- ☐ Increase to 20-25 minutes daily by Week 8
- ☐ Add stretching routine (5-10 minutes)
- ☐ Try gentle intervals if ready
- ☐ Listen to your body (back off if needed)

Social Navigation

- ☐ Successfully navigate one restaurant meal
- ☐ Attend one social event (party, potluck, gathering)
- ☐ Practice your response scripts
- ☐ Don't apologize for your choices

Tracking

Week #: ________________________________

New foods tried: ________________________________

Reactions (if any): ________________________________

Exercise minutes: ________________________________

Social situations handled: ________________________________

Biggest win: ________________________________

Biggest challenge: ________________________________

Coming Up:

Weeks 9-12 bring Phase 3—personalization, optimization, and the complete 90-day transformation. You'll fine-tune everything for YOUR body, test remaining triggers, and transition from protocol to lifestyle.

Elena will run her first 5K. Marcus will negotiate a four-day work week. James will teach his grandson to fish every weekend.

You've completed Weeks 5-8. You've expanded your variety, progressed your movement, and navigated the real world successfully.

You're not following someone else's rules anymore. You're making informed decisions based on YOUR body's responses.

That's mastery.

"Week 6 was when I realized restriction wasn't the goal. Freedom was. And I had more food freedom than I'd had in years." — Elena Martinez

"I ate at five different restaurants in three days and didn't have a single issue. This is actually sustainable." — Marcus Chen

"I tried foods I'd avoided for years. Most of them were fine. Should have tested sooner." — James Morrison

CHAPTER 8:

PHASE 2 CHECKPOINT & TRIGGER TESTING

Day 60: Three Transformations

Elena's Bathroom - Saturday Morning

Elena stood on the scale. 153 pounds. She'd started at 178.

Twenty-five pounds in sixty days.

But that wasn't what made her cry. It was the photo comparison on her phone. Day 1 Elena looked exhausted. Puffy face. Tired eyes. Shoulders slumped. She looked defeated.

Day 60 Elena looked alive.

She opened her tracking journal. Sixty days of data.

Pain levels:

Day 1	8/10 daily average
Day 30	3/10 daily average
Day 60	0-1/10 most days

Pain-free days:

Week 1	0
Week 4	12 out of 30
Week 8	27 out of 30

She'd had three minor pain spikes in the past month. Each traceable to a specific trigger: stress week, hidden sugar, three nights of poor sleep.

But no flares. No attacks. No days unable to walk.

Sofia knocked on the door. "Mom, are you crying?"

"Happy crying."

"Why?"

"Because I can run. Because I played tag with you last week and my toe didn't hurt. Because I'm training for a 5K. Because I feel like me again."

Sofia hugged her. "I like this version of you."

"Me too, kiddo. Me too."

Marcus's Doctor's Office - Friday Afternoon

Dr. Patel stared at the lab results. Then at Marcus. Then back at the screen.

"These can't be right."

"What's wrong?"

"Nothing's wrong. That's the problem." He pulled up the comparison. "Two months ago, your uric acid was 9.2. Today it's 6.1."

"Is that good?"

"That's excellent. That's optimal range." Dr. Patel scrolled through more results. "Your fasting glucose went from 142 to 94. Your A1C dropped from 7.1 to 5.8. You're no longer pre-diabetic."

Marcus felt his chest tighten. "What does that mean?"

"It means we're reducing your metformin. Possibly eliminating it if this holds. Your triglycerides dropped 95 points. Your CRP—your inflammation marker—went from 8.2 to 2.1."

"The inflammation is down?"

"Significantly. Marcus, in twenty years of practice, I've had maybe five patients reverse their metabolic syndrome trajectory. You're one of them."

They discussed medication adjustments. Metformin reduced by 50%. Blood pressure medication reduced. Check back in 30 days to potentially reduce further.

Marcus walked out and sat in his car for ten minutes.

Two months ago, he was limping at his daughter's wedding, on four medications, pre-diabetic, heading toward a heart attack like his father.

Today, he was reversing everything. Not managing. Reversing.

James's Garden - Friday Evening

James stood in his garden holding a fishing rod. Tyler was beside him, watching intently.

"Like this, Grandpa?"

"Exactly like that. Now flick your wrist—there! Perfect cast."

They were practicing for tomorrow's fishing trip. The real one. The one James had promised for a year. The one he thought he'd never be physically able to do.

Susan watched from the porch, wiping her eyes.

Later, after Tyler left, James showed Susan his lab results.

Kidney function:

Two months ago	eGFR 52, Creatinine 1.4
Today	eGFR 58, Creatinine 1.2

"Your kidneys improved," Susan said, staring at the numbers.

"The doctor said kidney function at my stage doesn't improve. He called me himself. Said he wanted to know exactly what I was doing."

James looked at his hands. "Sue, my hands don't hurt. I built that bird-house for Tyler last week. I'm working in the garden for hours without pain. I'm taking him fishing tomorrow and I'm not worried about whether I can do it. I know I can."

"How's your uric acid?"

"7.3. Not perfect, but down from 10.1. And I haven't had a flare in forty-three days."

Susan hugged him. "You did it, Jim."

"We did it. You did this with me every step."

Your 60-Day Complete Assessment

You've completed Phase 2. Sixty days. Two full months. Time to measure everything.

Physical Transformation
Weight and Body Composition:

Day 1 Weight:	
Day 60 Weight:	
Total Change:	

But more importantly:

- Compare Day 1 and Day 60 photos side by side
- How do your clothes fit?
- What do others say?

Pain Assessment:

Day 1 Average Pain: _____/10
Day 30 Average Pain: _____/10
Day 60 Average Pain: _____/10

Pain-free days:

Week 1-4: _____ out of 30
Week 5-8: _____ out of 30

Current status:

Completely pain-free? Y / N
Manageable pain only? Y / N
Better than Day 1? Y / N (should be yes)

Energy and Vitality:

Day 1 Average: _____/10
Day 60 Average: _____/10

Can you do these things now?

- Work full day without exhaustion
- Have energy for evening activities
- Exercise without depleting yourself
- Stay awake past 8 PM
- Wake up feeling rested
- Do activities you couldn't before

Sleep Quality:

Day 1: _____ hours, quality _____/10
Day 60: _____ hours, quality _____/10

Lab Results Comparison (If Available):

Uric Acid: _____ → _____
eGFR: _____ → _____
Fasting Glucose: _____ → _____
A1C: _____ → _____
CRP: _____ → _____
Blood Pressure: _____ → _____

Medication Changes (With Doctor Supervision)

Medications on Day 1:

1. ____________ (dose: _____)

2. ____________ (dose: _____)

Medications on Day 60:

1. ____________ (dose: _____)

2. ____________ (dose: _____)

What changed:

- Eliminated: ____________

- Reduced: ____________

Marcus reduced two medications by 50%. James eliminated one entirely. Both under doctor supervision.

Lifestyle Mastery

Check all that apply by Day 60:

☐ Meal prep is routine, not stressful
☐ Hydration is automatic
☐ Daily movement feels natural
☐ Restaurant ordering is confident
☐ Social situations navigated successfully
☐ Travel doesn't derail progress
☐ This feels sustainable long-term

The Mindset Transformation

Day 1, I believed: (Check what applied)

☐ My body is broken
☐ I'll always be in pain
☐ Change is too hard
☐ I'll fail like I always do

Day 60, I believe: (Check what applies now)

☐ My body can heal
☐ I have control
☐ Change is possible
☐ I can do hard things
☐ This is just how I live now

The identity shift:

Day 1: "I'm someone with gout trying to get better"
Day 60: "I'm someone who takes care of their health"

That shift is everything.

Introduction to Systematic Trigger Testing

You've been eating "safe" for sixty days. You know what definitely works. But you don't know your personal boundaries yet.

It's time to test systematically.

Why Test Triggers

Reason 1: Everyone is different
Elena can eat lentils without issues. Marcus can tolerate shrimp. James can eat mushrooms freely. All are on traditional "avoid" lists.

But Elena reacts to raw tomatoes. Marcus can't touch beer. James has issues with anything processed.

Reason 2: Knowledge is freedom
Right now, you're avoiding entire categories of foods "just in case." Long-term? You deserve to know exactly what YOU can and can't eat.

Reason 3: Empowerment
When you know your personal triggers, you make informed decisions instead of fearful ones.

What Not to Test

Never test:

- Processed sugar (we know this is inflammatory)
- Refined grains (same)
- Seed oils (same)
- Alcohol in large amounts (definitely triggers)

These are universal triggers. Save your testing energy for gray-area foods.

What to Test

Gray-area foods worth testing:
Higher-purine foods that might be okay:

- Shellfish (shrimp, scallops, crab)
- Specific fish (tuna, trout)
- Certain vegetables (asparagus, mushrooms, spinach—if you've been avoiding)
- Beans/lentils (if you've been avoiding)

Foods you miss:

- Moderate alcohol (one glass wine)
- Occasional higher-quality carb (sourdough bread, wild rice)
- Dairy (if you've been avoiding)

Foods in social situations:

- Wedding cake (one piece?)
- Birthday dinner (appetizer?)

Be strategic. Test things that matter to you.

The Testing Protocol

This is science. Treat it scientifically.

Step 1: Choose ONE Food to Test

Not three. Not "a meal with several new things." ONE food in isolation.

Example: Shrimp

Step 2: Establish Baseline

Three days before test:

- No new foods
- No unusual stress
- Normal sleep
- Normal exercise
- No pain or minimal pain (1-2/10 max)

Record baseline:

- Pain level: _____
- Energy level: _____
- Digestion: Normal / Good / Excellent
- Sleep last night: _____
- Stress level: _____

If you're having a flare, wait until it resolves.

Step 3: The Test

On test day:

- Eat the food in a moderate portion
- With an otherwise normal, safe meal
- At a normal time of day
- Under normal conditions (not during high stress)

Example: Grilled shrimp (6-8 pieces) with vegetables and quinoa at dinner.

Document:

- Food tested: _____________
- Portion size: _____________
- Time consumed: _____

- Other foods in meal: ____________
- Context (stress, sleep, etc.): ____________

Step 4: Monitor Carefully

Hour-by-hour tracking (first 12 hours):

2 hours after:

- Pain level: _____
- Digestion: _____
- Any symptoms: _____

6 hours after:

- Pain level: _____
- Any symptoms: _____

12 hours after (next morning):

- Pain level: _____
- Morning stiffness: _____
- Sleep quality: _____

24 hours after:

- Pain level: _____
- Any new symptoms: _____

48 hours after:

- Pain level: _____
- Full assessment: _____

72 hours after:

- Final pain level: _____
- Final assessment: _____

Step 5: Analyze Results

Clear negative reaction:

- Pain increased by 3+ points
- Joint swelling
- Redness/heat in joints
- Digestive upset

Verdict: AVOID this food

Mild reaction:

- Pain increased by 1-2 points
- Slight discomfort
- Minor digestive changes
- Resolved within 24 hours

Verdict: CAUTION - small amounts occasionally, or avoid

No reaction:

- Pain stayed same or decreased
- Energy good
- Digestion good
- Sleep good

Verdict: SAFE - add to regular rotation

Unclear result:

- Maybe something happened, maybe not
- Could have been other factors

Verdict: Test again in 2 weeks

Step 6: Wait Before Next Test
Minimum 5 days between tests
7 days is better

This ensures any delayed reaction has time to show and baseline is re-established.

Don't rush this process.

Real Testing Journeys

Marcus's Testing
Test 1: Shrimp (Day 62) Moderate portion at dinner. Watched carefully. No reaction. Added to safe list.

Test 2: Wine (Day 69) One glass red wine with dinner. Toe slightly swollen next morning (2/10 pain). Resolved by evening. Verdict: Caution. Very occasional only.

Test 3: Beer (Day 77) One beer. Toe painful within 4 hours (5/10). Swelling by morning. Clear reaction. Verdict: Absolutely avoid.

Test 4: White rice (Day 84) Small portion with stir-fry. No issues. Safe.

Conclusions:

- Shrimp: Fine
- Wine: Rare occasions only
- Beer: Never (his metabolism doesn't process it well)
- White rice: Moderate amounts okay

Marcus now knows his personal boundaries.

Elena's Testing

Test 1: Lentils (Day 63) Full serving in curry. No reaction. Safe list.

Test 2: Raw tomatoes (Day 70) Caprese salad with fresh mozzarella. Stomach upset within 2 hours. Mild pain increase (0 to 3/10). Resolved by next day. Verdict: Avoid raw. (Cooked tomatoes fine.)

Test 3: Mushrooms (Day 76) Large serving sautéed. No reaction. Safe list.

Test 4: Dark chocolate (Day 83) Small amount (2 squares 85% cacao). No issues. Safe list.

Conclusions:

- Lentils: Completely safe
- Raw tomatoes: Avoid (cooked fine)
- Mushrooms: Safe
- Dark chocolate: Safe in moderation

Elena expanded her diet significantly without triggering issues.

James's Testing

James's approach was simpler, less systematic, but effective.

Week 9: Tried beans in chili. Fine. Eats regularly now.

Week 10: Had processed deli meat. Toe hurt that evening. Avoided since.

Week 11: Tried one beer at church picnic. Pain by bedtime. Never again.

Week 12: Mushrooms in stir-fry. No issues. Eats from garden now.

James's conclusions:

- Real food: Fine
- Anything processed: Not fine

- Alcohol: Not fine
- Garden vegetables: All fine, even "high purine" ones

Simple rules that work for his life.

Recording Your Tests

Use this template for each test:

TRIGGER TEST LOG

Test Number: ____________
Date: ____________
Food Tested: ____________
Portion Size: ____________

Baseline (day before):

- Pain level: _____
- Energy: _____
- Sleep: _____
- Stress: _____

Tracking:

	Pain Level	Notes
+2 hours		
+6 hours		
+12 hours		
+24 hours		
+48 hours		

CONCLUSION:

☐ SAFE - Add to regular rotation
☐ CAUTION - Small amounts occasionally
☐ AVOID - Clear trigger
☐ UNCLEAR - Test again

Building Your Personal Food Lists

After 4-6 tests, you'll start seeing patterns.

Your GREEN LIGHT Foods (Safe - Eat Freely)

Proteins: ____________________

Vegetables: ____________________

Fats: ____________________

Carbs: ____________________

Your YELLOW LIGHT Foods (Caution - Occasional, Small Amounts)

Food: _____ **Frequency:** _____ **Portion limit:** ____

Your RED LIGHT Foods (Avoid - Clear Triggers)

1. ____________________
2. ____________________
3. ____________________

Patterns You've Noticed:

Foods/situations that consistently cause problems:

____

Foods you thought would be problems but aren't:

Surprising discoveries:

TAKE ACTION: Your 60-Day Checkpoint

Complete Assessment

- ☐ Take Day 60 photos
- ☐ Record all measurements
- ☐ Compare to Day 1 and Day 30
- ☐ Get lab work done (if haven't recently)
- ☐ List all non-scale victories

Trigger Testing Plan

Plan your next 4-6 tests:

	Trigger Test	Target Date
Test 1		
Test 2		
Test 3		
Test 4		

Space them 5-7 days apart.

Celebrate Phase 2 Completion

Before moving to Phase 3, celebrate:

Sixty days ago, you were in pain. Possibly on multiple medications. Probably skeptical this would work. Definitely uncertain you could sustain it.

Today, you're proof that transformation is possible.

You did this. Sixty days of showing up. Of making different choices. Of staying consistent even when it was hard.

Phase 3 brings you home. But Phase 2 proved you could do this in the real world.

Coming Up:

Phase 3 (Days 61-90) is about personalization, optimization, and making this permanent. You'll fine-tune everything for YOUR body and build the sustainable system you'll use long-term.

Elena will run that 5K. Marcus will negotiate his four-day work week. James will teach Tyler to fish every weekend.

Your story is just as important.

"Day 60 was when I stopped tracking to see if it was working and started tracking to understand my body better. I already knew it worked." — Elena Martinez

"My doctor said 'whatever you're doing, don't stop.' I realized I wouldn't stop even if he hadn't said it. This is just who I am now." — Marcus Chen

"Sixty days ago, I couldn't imagine teaching my grandson to fish. Tomorrow, we're going fishing. That's the only metric that matters." — James Morrison

---

CHAPTER 9:

WEEKS 9–10 – PERSONALIZING YOUR PROTOCOL

Day 61: Three New Beginnings

Elena's Kitchen - Sunday Afternoon

Elena stood at her counter with three cookbooks open, her laptop displaying a meal planning app, and Sofia beside her with a notebook.

"What are we doing?" Sofia asked.

"Creating our personal meal rotation. No more following someone else's plan. We're building ours."

For eight weeks, Elena had followed frameworks, templates, suggestions. She'd learned what worked. Now it was time to make it her own.

She pulled out her food journal. Sixty days of meals, annotated with notes. Green check marks next to meals they loved. Stars next to easy prep. Circles around budget-friendly. X's through things that didn't work.

"Okay, what do we actually like eating?" Elena asked.

Sofia started listing: "That lentil curry. The sheet pan chicken. The salmon with asparagus. Your turkey chilli. The stir-fry."

They spent an hour building their personal rotation. Not exotic recipes requiring specialty ingredients. Not complicated preparations. Just real food they actually enjoyed eating.

Elena's Weeknight Dinners (Rotation of 10):

1. Lentil curry (batch cook Sunday)
2. Sheet pan chicken and vegetables
3. Salmon with roasted asparagus
4. Turkey chilli (batch cook)
5. Stir-fry (rotating proteins)
6. Grilled chicken with quinoa and salad
7. Baked cod with Brussels sprouts

8. Ground turkey with vegetables
9. Chicken soup (batch cook)
10. Burrito bowl (no rice, extra vegetables)

Ten dinners. Rotate through them. Never bored because she actually liked all of them. Never stressed because she knew how to make them all.

“What about when we’re really tired?” Sofia asked.

“Leftovers. Or rotisserie chicken with bagged salad. Or eggs. We always have backup.”

Elena realized: personalization didn’t mean complicated. It meant choosing what worked for her life and letting go of what didn’t.

Marcus’s Home Office - Monday Morning

Marcus opened his spreadsheet. Not his work spreadsheet. His health optimization spreadsheet.

He’d tracked everything for nine weeks. Now he was analyzing patterns.

Best energy days: Correlate with 8+ hours sleep, morning exercise, no alcohol previous night

Worst energy days: Correlate with <7 hours sleep, skipped exercise, high stress

Best pain days (zero pain): Correlate with consistent hydration, stress management, regular sleep schedule

He looked at his meal data. Which foods made him feel best?

Post-meal energy ratings:

High energy meals:

- Salmon with vegetables and quinoa: 9/10

- Steak with large salad: 9/10
- Chicken stir-fry with lots of vegetables: 8/10

Low energy meals:

- Any meal with rice (even though blood sugar fine): 6/10
- Meals too large: 6/10

Marcus's body was teaching him. More protein and fat, moderate carbs from vegetables, gave him optimal energy. Rice, while not triggering gout, made him sleepy.

He created his personalized protocol:

Marcus's Non-Negotiables:

- Sleep: 11 PM - 7 AM (8 hours, non-negotiable)
- Exercise: 5:30 AM daily except Sunday
- Meals: Protein + vegetables + fat (heavy on protein)
- Hydration: 100 oz daily minimum
- Stress: 5-minute meditation morning, no email after 9 PM
- Alcohol: One glass wine max, once weekly, special occasions only

Marcus's Flexibility Points:

- Meal timing (as needed for schedule)
- Exercise type (as long as 30 minutes)
- Social situations (planned indulgences, back on track next meal)
- Travel adjustments (maintain principles, adjust execution)

This was his formula. Derived from data. Tested through experience. Optimized for his body and life.

Jennifer found him staring at his spreadsheet. "Still tracking?"

"Differently now. Not tracking to see if it works. Tracking to optimize what works."

"And?"

"I've figured out my formula. Sleep, exercise, protein-heavy meals, stress management. Do those things, I feel great. Skip them, I don't."

"That simple?"

"That simple. The data doesn't lie."

James's Garden - Monday Afternoon

James sat on his garden bench with a simple notebook. No spreadsheets. No apps. Just a list.

What Works for Me:

Food:

- Garden vegetables (unlimited)
- Fish (3-4 times per week)
- Chicken (daily if I want)
- Eggs (daily)
- Beans and lentils (turns out these are fine)
- Fruit (2-3 servings)
- No processed anything
- Quality over quantity

Movement:

- Garden work (1-2 hours most days)
- Morning stretches (10 minutes)
- Walking when it rains
- Fishing with Tyler (bonus movement)

Sleep:

- Bed by 9:30 PM
- Up by 6:00 AM
- That's 8.5 hours
- Feel best with this schedule

Stress:

- Garden time = stress relief
- Saying no to obligations I don't want
- Time with Tyler = best medicine
- Susan = everything

James looked at his list. It wasn't complicated. It was just life, structured around health.

He didn't need meal plans. He ate what came from his garden, plus protein from the store.

He didn't need workout schedules. He worked in his garden and played with his grandson.

He didn't need stress management techniques. He did things he loved and said no to things he didn't.

Susan came out. "What are you thinking about?"

"How simple this actually is. Eat real food. Move my body. Sleep enough. Do things I enjoy. Don't eat garbage or do things that stress me out."

"That's it?"

"That's it. I spent twelve years making it complicated. Turns out it's just living right."

Building Your Customized Meal Rotation

You've tried dozens of meals over nine weeks. Some you loved. Some were okay. Some you never want to make again.

Time to build your personal rotation from the winners.

The 3-Week Rotation System

Instead of the same seven meals every week (boring), create a three-week rotation with variety.

Week 1 Theme: Mediterranean
Week 2 Theme: Asian-Inspired
Week 3 Theme: American/Comfort

Then repeat. By the time you return to Week 1, it feels fresh again.

Elena's Approach: The Simple Rotation

Elena identified her five favorite proteins and five favorite preparations. Mix and match.

Proteins:

1. Chicken (breast or thigh)
2. Salmon
3. Ground turkey
4. Eggs
5. Lentils

Preparations:

1. Sheet pan roasted
2. Stir-fried
3. In soup/chilli
4. Grilled
5. Scrambled/in frittata

5 proteins × 5 preparations = 25 different meals

Add different vegetables each time. Add different spices. Suddenly you have endless variety from simple components.

Marcus's Approach: The Template System

Marcus built meal templates, not specific recipes.

Template 1: Protein + Green Vegetable + Salad

- Steak + asparagus + arugula salad
- Chicken + broccoli + mixed greens
- Salmon + green beans + spinach salad

Template 2: Protein + Roasted Vegetables + Grain

- Chicken + roasted peppers/onions + quinoa
- Fish + roasted Brussels sprouts + wild rice

Template 3: Bowl-Style

- Protein + cauliflower rice + vegetables + avocado + salsa

Template 4: Soup/Stew

- Protein + vegetables + broth + spices

Pick a template. Choose proteins and vegetables based on what's available. Never think too hard about it.

James's Approach: Seasonal and Simple

James's rotation followed his garden's output.

Spring: Asparagus, lettuce, radishes, peas
Summer: Tomatoes, peppers, zucchini, cucumbers

Fall: Brussels sprouts, kale, squash, carrots
Winter: Stored root vegetables, frozen from summer

Add protein from store (fish, chicken, eggs). That's the meal.

No recipes needed. If it grows in your garden and it's healthy, eat it with protein.

Your Personal Plate Formula

By now, you know what your body needs. Time to formalize it.

Elena's Personal Formula
Breakfast: Protein + healthy fat + some carbs

- Example: Eggs + avocado + berries

Lunch: Protein + lots of vegetables + light carb

- Example: Chicken + large salad + small portion quinoa

Dinner: Protein + 2-3 different vegetables + optional carb

- Example: Salmon + asparagus + salad + small sweet potato

Portions:

- Protein: palm-sized
- Vegetables: unlimited
- Carbs: fist-sized or smaller
- Fats: thumb-sized

Marcus's Personal Formula

Marcus discovered he does best with higher protein, moderate fat, lower carbs.

Every meal:

- 40% protein
- 30% vegetables
- 20% healthy fats
- 10% carbs (from vegetables mostly)

No snacks (meals keep him full enough)

Hydration: 100 oz minimum, more on exercise days

James's Personal Formula

James learned his body does well with simplicity and quality.

Every meal: Real food, mostly plants, some quality protein

Breakfast: Eggs + vegetables from garden + fruit
Lunch: Last night's dinner
Dinner: Fish or chicken + garden vegetables (2-3 kinds) + beans occasionally

Portions: Eat until satisfied, not stuffed. Stop when 80% full.

Non-negotiables:

- Nothing processed
- Nothing from a box with more than 5 ingredients
- Vegetables at every meal
- Real butter, real olive oil (no fake fats)

Creating Flexibility Within Structure

You need structure for consistency. You need flexibility for sustainability.

The 80/20 Framework

80% of the time: Follow your personal protocol strictly
20% of the time: Planned flexibility

What 80/20 does NOT mean:

- 20% junk food
- 20% going back to old patterns
- 20% "cheat days"

What 80/20 DOES mean:

- 20% special occasions (weddings, birthdays, holidays)
- 20% controlled indulgences (one glass wine, small dessert)
- 20% flexibility in timing, preparation, or food choices
- 20% "good enough" instead of "perfect"

Elena's 80/20:

- 80%: Home-cooked meals from her rotation
- 20%: Restaurants, date nights, Sofia's birthday party, occasional pizza night

Marcus's 80/20:

- 80%: Strict protocol, especially weekdays
- 20%: Weekend dinners out, business meals, special occasions

James's 80/20:

- 80%: Garden food + simple proteins
- 20%: Church potlucks, family gatherings, Tyler's birthday

Planned Indulgences vs. Unplanned Slip-Ups

Planned indulgence: Wedding cake (one piece), enjoyed, no guilt, back to normal next meal

Unplanned slip-up: Stress-ate a bag of chips, felt terrible, took 2 days to get back on track

One is strategic. One is reactive.

Make indulgences planned:

- Know in advance
- Decide parameters (one glass wine, not three)
- Enjoy fully without guilt
- Return to protocol immediately after
- Don't let one meal become one day become one week

When slip-ups happen (they will):

- No guilt or shame
- Get back on track next meal (not tomorrow, not Monday, NEXT MEAL)
- Analyze what triggered it
- Create strategy to prevent it
- Move on

Your Personal "Safe Foods" List

After nine weeks and several trigger tests, you know your safe foods.

Building Your Lists

My Green Light Foods (Eat Freely):

Group	Food
Proteins	
Vegetables	
Health Fats	
Carbs	

My Yellow Light Foods (Occasional, Small Amounts):

Food	Frequency	Portion	Conditions

My Red Light Foods (Never):

Food	Reason

Your Personal Planning System

Elena's Weekly Planning

Sunday:

- Review calendar for week
- Identify busy days vs. normal days
- Choose 5-7 dinners from rotation
- Make grocery list
- Shop
- Batch cook 1-2 items
- Prep vegetables for week

Daily:

- Morning: pack lunch (leftovers or salad with protein)
- Dinner: one of planned meals (20-30 minutes)

Time investment: 3 hours Sunday, 20-30 min daily

Marcus's Template Approach

No weekly planning. Just templates and stocked fridge.

Always in fridge:

- Proteins (chicken, fish, steak)
- Greens (multiple types)
- Vegetables (5-6 kinds)
- Quinoa or rice (pre-cooked in batches)
- Hard-boiled eggs

At mealtime:

- Pick a template
- Choose protein and vegetables
- Cook (15-30 minutes)

Time investment: 1 hour grocery shopping weekly, 15-30 min per meal

James's Seasonal Simplicity

Planning: Walk through garden, see what's ready

Meal: Pick vegetables, choose protein from fridge, cook together

Time investment: Minimal. Garden time counts as both food production and exercise.

All three systems work. Pick what fits your life.

TAKE ACTION: Build Your Personal System

Create Your Meal Rotation
List your 10 favorite meals from the past 9 weeks:

1. ______________________________
2. ______________________________
3. ______________________________
4. ______________________________
5. ______________________________
6. ______________________________
7. ______________________________
8. ______________________________
9. ______________________________
10. ______________________________

These form your base rotation.

Define Your Personal Formula

My ideal breakfast: ____________
My ideal lunch: ____________
My ideal dinner: ____________

My portion sizes:

- Protein: ____________
- Vegetables: ____________
- Carbs: ____________
- Fats: ____________

Set Your Boundaries

My 80%: ____________
My 20%: ____________
My green light foods: ____________
My yellow light foods: ____________
My red light foods: ____________

Create Your Planning System

My meal planning approach: (Weekly plan / Template system / Seasonal simplicity / Other)

My shopping day: ____________
My prep day: ____________
My time investment: ____________

Coming Up:

Weeks 11-12 bring advanced optimization—fine-tuning supplement timing, exercise intensity, stress management depth. The final polish before Day 90.

But the personalization you've done in Weeks 9-10? This is the foundation of your permanent lifestyle.

You're not following the protocol anymore. The protocol has become you.

"I stopped trying to eat like someone else and started eating like the healthiest version of me. Turns out, she likes simple food that tastes good." — Elena Martinez

"Data revealed my formula: sleep 8 hours, exercise 30 minutes, eat mostly protein and vegetables, manage stress. Deviation from formula equals deviation from results." — Marcus Chen

"Complex plans fail. Simple plans sustained with discipline succeed. Garden food + quality protein + movement + rest = health." — James Morrison

---

CHAPTER 10:

WEEKS 11-12 - ADVANCED OPTIMIZATION

Day 75: Three Peaks

Elena's Morning - 5K Race Day

Elena stood at the starting line surrounded by hundreds of runners. Sofia was beside her, bouncing with nervous energy.

"You ready, Mom?"

Elena looked down at her running bib. Number 2847. Three months ago, she could barely walk without pain. Today, she was running a 5K.

The gun fired. They started moving.

Mile 1: She felt strong. Breathing controlled. Legs good. No pain anywhere.

Mile 2: Sofia was chatting beside her. Elena was still comfortable. This was actually... fun?

Mile 3: The finish line appeared. Sofia grabbed her hand. "Let's finish together!"

They crossed at 34 minutes, 12 seconds. Not fast. But they finished. Running.

Elena's eyes filled with tears. She'd done it. The goal she set on Day 47 when the idea seemed impossible.

Sofia hugged her. "Mom, you're crying again."

"Happy crying. Always happy crying now."

That afternoon, Elena reviewed her training data. Twelve weeks of progressive building without a single flare. Her body had adapted. Not just to running, but to being healthy.

She'd optimized everything: hydration timing around runs, meal timing for energy, sleep schedule for recovery, stress management to prevent overtraining. The 5K was just the visible result. The optimization was the real achievement.

Marcus's Office - Thursday Evening

Marcus sat across from his boss, Tom.

"I'm cutting back to four days a week starting next quarter."

Tom blinked. "Marcus, you're VP of Operations. That's not really—"

"I know. And I'm still doing the job. Just compressed into four days instead of five."

"Why?"

Marcus had prepared for this. "Two months ago, my doctor told me I was reversing metabolic syndrome. First time in his twenty-year career he's seen it happen this dramatically. You want to know how?"

Tom nodded.

"I sleep eight hours. I exercise thirty minutes every morning. I manage my stress. I spend time with my wife. And I realized that cramming all that into weekends while working sixty-hour weeks was killing me. Literally."

"And four days works?"

"I've been testing it. I'm more productive in four focused days than I was in five distracted ones. Better decisions. More energy. No burnout."

Tom was quiet. Then: "Your results have been excellent lately."

"Because I'm healthy. Healthy Marcus is better at his job than sick Marcus ever was."

"Okay. Four days. But this is an experiment."

"Agreed. And if my results decline, we revisit."

They didn't decline. Marcus had optimized his entire life. Work was just one component.

James's Boat - Saturday Morning

James and Tyler sat in the boat, lines in the water, sun rising.

Tyler had caught two bass. James had caught three. They'd been out since 6 AM.

"Grandpa, are we going to do this every week?"

"If you want to."

"I want to."

James looked at his grandson. This moment—this exact moment—was why he'd committed to the protocol eleven weeks ago.

At the birthday party, he couldn't get on the floor. Now he was in a boat, fishing, teaching his grandson, no pain anywhere in his body.

They fished until noon. James's back was tired but not screaming. His knees were stiff but functional. His hands worked the fishing line without cramping.

On the drive home, Tyler fell asleep. James looked at him in the rearview mirror.

"Thank you," James said to no one in particular. To his body for healing. To Susan for supporting him. To whatever made him finally commit to change.

That evening, Susan found him in the garden.

"Good day?"

"Best day. We're doing it again next Saturday."

"Your body holding up okay?"

"Better than okay. I feel..." James searched for the word. "Young. Not 25 young. But like I have years ahead of me instead of just getting through today."

Susan kissed his cheek. "You do have years ahead of you. Many of them."

Advanced Hydration Strategies

By Week 11, basic hydration is automatic. Time to optimize.

Activity-Based Adjustments

Exercise days: Add 16-24 oz

- 8-12 oz before exercise
- Sip during if longer than 30 minutes
- 8-12 oz within 30 minutes after

Hot weather: Add 16-32 oz

- Sweat loss needs replacing
- Monitor urine color closely

Travel days: Add 16 oz

- Airplanes dehydrate
- More walking than usual

High-stress days: Add 8-16 oz

- Stress affects fluid retention
- Extra hydration helps

Electrolyte Optimization

Plain water isn't always enough, especially with higher activity.

Signs you need more electrolytes:

- Drinking plenty but still thirsty
- Light-headedness when standing
- Muscle cramps
- Fatigue despite adequate water

How to add electrolytes:
Option 1: Food sources (best)

- Sea salt in meals
- Leafy greens (potassium, magnesium)
- Avocados (potassium)
- Nuts and seeds (magnesium)

Option 2: Add to water

- Pinch of sea salt per liter
- Squeeze of lemon (potassium)
- Unsweetened coconut water

Marcus added a pinch of sea salt to his morning lemon water and post-exercise water. Made significant difference in energy and recovery.

Timing Optimization

Morning hydration (critical):

- 16 oz within 30 minutes of waking
- With lemon and pinch of salt
- Before coffee
- Kickstarts everything

Pre-meal hydration:

- 8-12 oz about 15-20 minutes before meals
- Aids digestion
- Helps with satiety

Exercise timing:

- Before: 8-12 oz (30 min prior)
- During: Sip as needed (if >30 min)
- After: 8-12 oz (within 30 min)

Evening taper:

- Last large glass 2 hours before bed
- Small sips only closer to bedtime
- Reduces nighttime bathroom trips

Supplement Timing Optimization

You've been taking supplements (hopefully). Now optimize timing for maximum benefit.

Evidence-Based Supplements

What likely helps:
Vitamin C (500-1000mg daily)

- Timing: With breakfast
- Why: Helps kidneys excrete uric acid

Omega-3 (2000-3000mg EPA+DHA)

- Timing: With largest meal
- Why: Anti-inflammatory, needs fat for absorption

Vitamin D (2000-5000 IU)

- Timing: With breakfast (fatty meal)
- Why: Immune function, inflammation control
- Note: Get levels tested first

Magnesium (300-400mg)

- Timing: Evening, 1 hour before bed
- Why: Aids sleep, muscle relaxation
- Best form: Glycinate (most absorbable)

Marcus's Supplement Stack (Data-Driven)
Morning (with breakfast):

- Vitamin C: 1000mg
- Omega-3: 2000mg
- Vitamin D: 4000 IU (his tested level was low)

Evening (before bed):

- Magnesium glycinate: 400mg

Total cost: ~$40/month

Results: Tracked for 4 weeks on vs. 2 weeks off. Noticed better recovery during off period. Resumed.

Elena's Minimal Approach
Morning:

- Multivitamin (covers basics)
- Omega-3

Evening:

- Magnesium (for sleep)

Her philosophy: Get most nutrients from food, supplement only gaps.

James's Even Simpler Approach
Morning:

- Vitamin D (doctor recommended for deficiency)

That's it. Everything else from garden vegetables, fish, and sunshine.

His philosophy: If great-grandparents didn't need it, he probably doesn't either.

All three approaches work. More supplements isn't better. Targeted supplementation based on YOUR needs is optimal.

Exercise Intensity Progression

Week 11-12 is about testing your capacity safely.

The 10% Rule Continues

Still increase by no more than 10% weekly. But now you're at higher baseline.

Week 11: 28 minutes daily average
Week 12: 30-31 minutes daily average

Or increase intensity while maintaining duration.

For Those Ready: Interval Training

What it is: Alternating higher and lower intensity

Why it works:

- Improves cardiovascular fitness faster
- Burns more calories in less time
- Builds metabolic flexibility
- Doesn't increase injury risk if done properly

Elena's Running Intervals:

- 5 min warm-up walk
- 2 min jog, 1 min walk (repeat 5x)
- 5 min cool-down walk
- Total: 25 minutes

Marcus's Walking Intervals:

- 5 min moderate pace
- 2 min fast pace (still walking, just faster)
- 3 min recovery pace
- Repeat 4x
- 5 min cool-down
- Total: 30 minutes

Key: The "hard" intervals shouldn't be that hard. You should be able to maintain conversation, just breathlessly.

Strength Training Progression

If you've been doing bodyweight exercises, time to add challenge.

Option 1: Increase reps

- Wall push-ups: 15 → 20
- Sit-to-stands: 15 → 20
- Holds: 30 seconds → 45 seconds

Option 2: Increase difficulty

- Wall push-ups → Counter push-ups → Floor push-ups (on knees)
- Sit-to-stands → Squats (no chair)
- Plank on knees → Plank on toes

Option 3: Add resistance

- Resistance bands (light to start)
- Light dumbbells (5-10 lbs)
- Household items (water bottles, cans)

Marcus's Week 11 routine:

- Push-ups (floor, on knees): 15 reps
- Squats (bodyweight): 20 reps
- Resistance band rows: 15 reps
- Plank (on knees): 45 seconds
- Repeat circuit 3x
- Total: 20 minutes

Still no gym required.

Stress Management Mastery

By Week 11, you have basic stress management. Time to deepen.

Beyond Basics

You're already doing:

- Recognizing stress
- Some form of daily practice
- Evening boundaries
- Sleep prioritization

Next level:

1. Anticipatory stress management

Don't wait until you're stressed. Prevent stress escalation.

Marcus's approach:

- Knows Monday mornings are stressful
- Does extra 5 minutes meditation Sunday night
- Goes to bed 30 minutes earlier Sunday
- Protects Monday morning from meetings
- Result: Monday stress reduced 60%

2. Stress as data, not enemy

Stress tells you something needs addressing.

Elena's reframe:

- Stress about money → addressed by budget review
- Stress about time → addressed by better boundaries
- Stress about daughter → addressed by dedicated time together

Solving root causes beats managing symptoms.

3. Physical stress release

James's discovery: Garden work as active meditation
Marcus's practice: Hard exercise when stressed (within safe limits)
Elena's method: Dance party with Sofia when stressed

Physical movement processes stress hormones.

Advanced Meditation Practice

If you've been doing 5 minutes, consider increasing to 10-15.

Why:

- Deeper relaxation response
- Better stress resilience
- Improved focus
- Lower baseline cortisol

Marcus's progression:

- Week 1-4: Resistant, didn't do it
- Week 5-6: 5 minutes daily (reluctantly)
- Week 7-8: 5 minutes (less resistant)
- Week 9-10: 8 minutes (actually helpful)
- Week 11-12: 10 minutes (non-negotiable)

His current practice:

- 5:15 AM (before exercise)
- Sit comfortably
- Focus on breath
- When mind wanders (constantly), return to breath
- No judgment
- Timer ends practice

Result: Completely changed his stress response and decision-making.

Sleep Optimization Deep Dive

You're sleeping better. Can you optimize further?

Sleep Tracking Analysis

If you've been tracking sleep:

Review last 30 days:

- Best sleep nights: What was common?
- Worst sleep nights: What preceded them?

Common patterns:

Better sleep correlates with:

- Exercise that day (but not within 3 hours of bed)
- No alcohol
- Screen cutoff 1+ hours before bed
- Consistent bedtime
- Cooler room (65-68°F)
- Stress managed earlier in day

Worse sleep correlates with:

- Skipped exercise
- Alcohol (even small amounts)
- Screens before bed
- Inconsistent schedule
- Hot room
- Unresolved stress
- Large meal too close to bedtime

The Perfect Evening Routine (Personalized)

Elena's evolved routine:

- 7:30 PM: Last screen time for work
- 8:00 PM: Light cleaning, prep for tomorrow
- 8:30 PM: Time with Sofia (talking, reading, no screens)
- 9:00 PM: Personal time (reading, bath, stretching)
- 9:30 PM: Bed (reads physical book)
- 10:00 PM: Lights out

Marcus's routine:

- 8:00 PM: Last work email
- 8:30 PM: Walk with Jennifer
- 9:00 PM: Shower, prepare for next day
- 9:30 PM: Reading or talking with Jennifer
- 10:00 PM: Magnesium supplement
- 10:30 PM: Lights out

James's routine:

- 8:00 PM: Evening stretches
- 8:30 PM: Sit on porch with Susan (no agenda)
- 9:00 PM: Prepare for bed, read
- 9:30 PM: Lights out

All different. All effective. Build what works for YOU.

The Final Polish

Week 11-12 is about removing final obstacles to optimal health.

What's Still Not Optimal?

Honest assessment:

Pain: Completely gone | Minimal | Still significant
Energy: Excellent | Good | Could be better
Sleep: Perfect | Good | Needs work
Stress: Well-managed | Okay | Still struggling
Weight: At goal | Close | Still working on it
Labs: Optimal | Good | Improving but not there yet

For each "could be better" or "needs work":

What's the obstacle? ______________________________
What haven't I tried? ______________________________
What could I optimize? ______________________________

Marcus's energy was "good" but not "excellent." He realized he needed more carbs around exercise. Added small sweet potato post-workout. Energy became excellent.

Elena's sleep was "good" but not "perfect." She was scrolling phone in bed. Removed phone from bedroom entirely. Sleep became perfect.

James's weight loss had plateaued. He realized portion sizes had crept up. Returned to conscious portions. Weight loss resumed.

Small optimizations, significant results.

Week 11-12 Goals and Milestones

Week 11: Fine-Tuning

Goals:

- Optimize one area that's "good but could be better"
- Test higher exercise intensity safely
- Review all supplement timing
- Identify any remaining obstacles

Elena's Week 11:

- Tested running intervals (success)
- Removed phone from bedroom (sleep improved)
- Reviewed supplement stack (added evening magnesium)
- Identified obstacle: occasional stress eating (created new strategy)

Week 12: Final Push

Goals:

- Prove you can maintain everything for full week perfectly
- Complete any remaining trigger tests
- Finalize your personal protocol
- Prepare for Day 90 assessment

Marcus's Week 12:

- Executed perfect week (all workouts, all meals, sleep, stress management)
- Completed wine trigger test (confirmed: caution category)
- Finalized four-day work week plan
- Prepared for Day 90 labs

TAKE ACTION: Your Optimization Checklist

Identify Optimization Opportunities

Rate these areas (1-10):

Nutrition: ______________________________

Hydration: ______________________________

Movement: ______________________________

Sleep: ______________________________

Stress Management: ______________________________

Pain Levels: ______________________________

Energy Levels: ______________________________

For any rated 7 or below, what's one thing you could optimize?

This Week's Experiments

Choose 1-2 to test:

- Increase exercise intensity slightly
- Optimize supplement timing
- Deepen meditation practice
- Perfect evening routine
- Test remaining trigger foods
- Address remaining obstacle

Week 12 Challenge

Execute one perfect week:

- Every planned workout completed
- Every meal on protocol
- Sleep 7-8 hours nightly
- Stress managed daily
- Hydration targets hit
- No unplanned indulgences

Can you do it? Prove to yourself you've mastered this.

Coming Up:

Chapter 15 covers your sustainable maintenance plan—how to keep this going beyond Day 90. Chapter 16 will be your complete 90-day review.

But first, finish strong. Week 12 is your victory lap.

You've already won. Now enjoy it.

"The 5K wasn't the goal. It was proof that I'd built a body capable of doing things I thought were impossible." — Elena Martinez

"Optimization isn't about perfection. It's about removing the obstacles between where you are and where you're capable of being." — Marcus Chen

"I didn't optimize for performance. I optimized for longevity. I want to fish with my great-grandchildren someday." — James Morrison

---

CHAPTER 11:

YOUR SUSTAINABLE MAINTENANCE PLAN

Day 85: Three Conversations

Elena's Coffee Shop - Saturday Morning

Elena sat across from Maria, who'd been part of the walking group since Week 2.

"So what happens after Day 90?" Maria asked. "Do you just... stop?"

Elena laughed. "Stop what? Living this way? No. This is just who I am now."

"But the protocol ends at 90 days."

"The protocol was the training wheels. Teaching me how to live healthy. But I'm not following a protocol anymore. I'm just living."

Maria looked worried. "What if you gain the weight back?"

"Then I deal with it. But Maria, I feel better than I have in ten years. I can run. I have energy. I'm not in pain. Why would I go back?"

"Most people do."

"Most people treat it like a diet with an end date. I treated it like building a new life. There's no end date to my life."

Elena pulled out her phone. "I'm not stopping at Day 90. I'm just moving from building phase to maintenance phase."

"What's the difference?"

"Building phase: learning, testing, tracking everything obsessively. Maintenance phase: living what I've learned, tracking occasionally, adjusting when needed."

"And you think you can maintain this forever?"

"Forever is too big. I can maintain this today. And tomorrow. That's all I need to think about."

Marcus's Kitchen - Sunday Evening

Marcus and Jennifer were cooking dinner together. Something they did every weekend now.

"What happens when the 90 days end?" Jennifer asked.

"Nothing changes."

"Really? You're not going to relax the rules?"

"What rules? These aren't rules. This is just how I eat now."

Marcus plated grilled chicken and vegetables. "Day 1 Marcus saw this as restriction. Day 85 Marcus sees this as freedom. The way I get to live."

"When did that shift happen?"

"Around Week 8, I stopped thinking 'I can't have that.' Started thinking 'I don't want that.' By Week 10, this stopped being effort. It became default."

"And work? The four-day schedule?"

"That's maintenance too. I proved I can do the job in four days. Why would I go back to five?"

Jennifer kissed him. "What if you slip up?"

"Then I slip up. One meal doesn't define me. The pattern defines me. And my pattern is solid."

James's Porch - Sunday Evening

James and Susan sat watching the sunset.

"Tyler asked if we're going fishing every Saturday forever," James said.

"What did you tell him?"

"As long as my body lets me. And I plan to make sure my body lets me for a very long time."

Susan took his hand. "You've changed. Not just your body. You."

"You're present now. Before, you were just surviving. Now you're living."

James nodded. "Twelve years of decline will do that. You forget what feeling good feels like. Then when you remember, you never want to forget again."

"Are you worried about Day 90?"

"No. Day 90 is just Saturday. I'll wake up, stretch, eat breakfast, work in the garden, maybe fish with Tyler. Same as Day 89. Same as Day 91."

"No celebration?"

"Every day I wake up without pain is a celebration."

Transitioning from Protocol to Lifestyle

The 90-Day Protocol isn't a diet that ends. It's a training program that teaches you how to live.

What Changes After Day 90
What DOESN'T change:

- Core nutrition principles
- Daily movement
- Adequate sleep
- Stress management
- Hydration

What DOES change:

- Intensity of tracking (daily → weekly or as-needed)

- Rigidity of schedule (more flexibility)
- Mental energy required (less, it's automatic)
- Identity (you're not "doing" this, you ARE this)

The shift:

Days 1-30: Following a protocol (effort required)
Days 31-60: Integrating (getting easier)
Days 61-90: Living it (mostly automatic)
Day 91+: Being it (just who you are)

The 80/20 Maintenance Approach
80% of the time: Your Protocol

- Monday-Friday: Strict adherence
- Home meals: Always on protocol
- Regular routine: Healthy defaults

20% of the time: Strategic Flexibility

- Special occasions (weddings, holidays)
- Social situations (restaurants, travel)
- Planned indulgences (conscious choices, no guilt)

What 80/20 does NOT mean:

- 20% junk food binge
- "Cheat days"
- Pendulum swinging between restriction and abandon

Real Examples
Elena's 80/20:

- 80%: Weekday meals, home dinners
- 20%: Date nights, Sofia's events, occasional treats

Marcus's 80/20:

- 80%: Monday-Thursday strict protocol
- 20%: Friday dinners, business meals, quarterly celebrations

James's 80/20:

- 80%: Garden vegetables, quality protein daily
- 20%: Church potlucks, Tyler's birthday, Thanksgiving

The Maintenance Tracking System

You don't need obsessive tracking. You need awareness.

Daily Tracking (Minimal)
Required daily (1 minute total):

- Pain level (0-10)
- Energy level (0-10)
- Sleep hours

That's it.

Weekly Check-Ins (10 minutes)

Every Sunday:
Review:

- Average pain: _____
- Average energy: _____
- Days exercised: _____
- Successes: _____
- Struggles: _____

Plan:

- Special events this week?
- Scheduled indulgences?
- Travel/disruptions?

Adjust:

- If pain increased: What changed?
- If energy decreased: What changed?
- If everything's great: Keep going

Monthly Deep Dive (30 minutes)

First Sunday of month:
Compare to last month:

- Pain trends
- Energy trends
- Weight trends
- Exercise consistency

Identify patterns:

- What's working well?
- What's sliding?
- What needs focus?

Set intentions:

- One area to optimize
- One area to maintain

Quarterly Assessments

Every 3 months:

- Full measurements
- Photos
- Lab work (annually minimum)
- Life quality reflection

Not obsessive. Just aware.

Strategic Indulgences

Indulgences happen. Make them strategic.

The Framework

Before:

1. Decide in advance ("I will have one piece of cake")
2. Set boundaries (One glass wine, not three)
3. Plan return (Next meal = protocol)

During:

1. Enjoy fully (No guilt)
2. Stay present (Eat slowly)
3. Honor boundaries (One means one)

After:

1. Return immediately (Very next meal)
2. No compensation (Don't skip meals)
3. Learn (Was it worth it?)

When It Goes Wrong

Marcus's business dinner: Stressed, exhausted. Had two wines, bread, dessert. Toe sore next morning.

His response: Immediately back on protocol. Extra hydration. Normal by day 3.

His learning: Stress + exhaustion + alcohol = bad for him. No indulgences during high-stress periods.

Preventing Backsliding

The risk isn't one indulgence. It's the slow slide.

Warning Signs

Physical:

- Pain creeping back
- Energy declining
- Weight climbing (5+ pounds)

Behavioral:

- Skipping exercise often
- Forgetting meal prep
- Reaching for processed foods

Mental:

- "I deserve this" replacing "is this worth it"
- Ignoring warning signs
- Losing sight of why

If you notice 3+, you're sliding.

Emergency Reset

When you're sliding:

1. **Acknowledge** ("I'm sliding. That's okay. Now I fix it.")
2. **Return to Phase 1 for 1 week** (Basic protocol, daily tracking)
3. **Identify what changed** (Stress? Circumstances? Boredom?)
4. **Address root cause** (If stress → stress management. If boredom → add variety)
5. **Create prevention strategy** (What will you do differently?)

Elena's reset: Week 30 post-program, eating out too much. One week Phase 1. Back on track.

Annual Tune-Up

Once yearly: Phase 1 for 2 weeks

Why:

- Resets drifted habits
- Reminds you how good you can feel
- Clears inflammation
- Refreshes motivation

When: Pick annual date (New Year, birthday, protocol anniversary)

What: Strict Phase 1, no indulgences, extra tracking, labs, photos

Benefits: Reset, comparison data, renewed commitment

Your Support System

Types of Support Needed

Accountability: Someone who knows your goals, calls you out lovingly

Knowledge: Healthcare providers who support this, community doing similar

Social: Friends/family who understand, activities supporting healthy lifestyle

Professional (if needed): Functional medicine doctor, nutritionist, therapist

When to Help Others

You're ready when:

- You've maintained 6+ months
- You have clear results
- You've handled setbacks
- You have time and energy

You're not ready if:

- Still figuring it out yourself
- Barely maintaining
- Want validation more than to help

How to help:

- Share when asked
- Offer specific strategies
- Be honest about challenges
- Support without pushing

Elena started helping around Month 6. Marcus waited until Month 12. James helps when asked but doesn't seek it out.

Your Personal Maintenance Formula

Document what maintains YOUR health:

My Non-Negotiables:

Foods I eat regularly: ____________________
Foods I never eat: ____________________
Daily habits: ____________________

My Flexibility Points:

Where I allow flexibility: ____________________
Boundaries within flexibility: ____________________

My Warning Signs:

If these happen, I'm sliding: ____________________

My Reset Protocol:

When sliding: ____________________

My Support System:

Accountability: ____________________
Healthcare team: ____________________
Social support: ____________________

The Truth About Forever

Forever is too big. Focus on today.

Can you maintain this today? Yes.
Tomorrow? Probably.

Next week? Likely.

Forever? Don't think about forever.

Think about:

- This meal
- This day
- This week

String enough successful days together, and forever takes care of itself.

Elena doesn't think about maintaining for life. She thinks about packing tomorrow's lunch.

Marcus doesn't worry about the next decade. He focuses on tonight's sleep.

James doesn't stress about forever. He plans this week's garden work.

One day at a time. That's the only sustainable approach.

TAKE ACTION: Build Your Maintenance Plan

Design Your Tracking System

What I'll track daily: ______________________________

What I'll review weekly: ______________________________

What I'll assess monthly: ______________________________

Quarterly check-ins: ______________________________

Plan Your First Strategic Indulgence

Upcoming event: ______________________________

Date: ______________________________

My plan:

- What I'll indulge in: ______________________
- My boundaries: ______________________
- My return plan: ______________________

Create Your Reset Protocol

If I notice sliding, I will:

1. ______________________
2. ______________________
3. ______________________

I will schedule my annual tune-up for: ______________________

Coming Up:

Chapter 16 is your complete 90-day review—the comprehensive comparison, the celebration, the complete transformation story.

Day 90 isn't the end. It's not even the beginning of the end. It's the end of the beginning.

The protocol taught you how to live. Now you live it.

Not perfectly. Not rigidly. Not obsessively.

Just healthily. Sustainably. Joyfully.

That's the maintenance plan. Not a plan at all. Just a life.

"Maintenance isn't maintaining perfection. It's maintaining awareness, making adjustments, and choosing health more often than not." — Elena Martinez

"The protocol ends at Day 90. The lifestyle never ends. That's not burden. That's freedom." — Marcus Chen

"I don't maintain this protocol. I live this life. There's a difference." — James Morrison

CHAPTER 12:

THE COMPLETE 90-DAY REVIEW

Day 90: Three Celebrations

Elena's Living Room - Friday Evening

Elena sat on her couch with her laptop open, looking at the photos she'd taken on Day 1. She barely recognized herself.

Not just the physical changes—though those were obvious. The puffy face was gone. The tired eyes were brighter. But it was something else. The woman in the Day 1 photos looked defeated. Resigned. Like she'd given up.

The woman looking back at her from the mirror now? She looked alive.

Sofia walked in. "Are you looking at your before pictures again?"

"How did you know?"

"Because you've looked at them like five times this week." Sofia sat next to her. "You look so different now."

"I lost twenty-five pounds."

"That's not what I mean." Sofia struggled to articulate it. "You look... lighter. Not weight lighter. Like, happier lighter. Does that make sense?"

Elena pulled up her tracking journal. Ninety days of data.

Day 1 pain level: 8/10
Day 90 pain level: 0-1/10

Day 1 energy level: 3/10
Day 90 energy level: 8/10

Days with flares: 0 in the past three weeks

Days exercised: 28 out of 30 last month

Meals prepped at home: 87 out of 90 last month

She'd done it. Ninety days. She'd actually stuck with something.

"Mom, are you crying?"

"I'm just proud of myself."

Sofia hugged her. "I'm proud of you too."

Marcus's Doctor's Office - Thursday Afternoon

Dr. Patel stared at the lab results on his screen. Then at Marcus. Then back at the screen.

"These can't be right."

"What's wrong?"

"Nothing's wrong. That's the problem. These numbers are too good." He pulled up the comparison screen. "Your uric acid went from 9.2 to 6.1. Your fasting glucose from 142 to 94. Your A1C dropped from 7.1 to 5.8. You're no longer pre-diabetic."

Marcus felt his chest tighten. "What does that mean?"

"It means we're reducing your metformin. Possibly eliminating it if this holds. Your triglycerides dropped 95 points. Your CRP—your inflammation marker—went from 8.2 to 2.1."

"The inflammation is down?"

"By 75%. Marcus, in twenty years of practice, I've had maybe five patients reverse their metabolic syndrome trajectory. You're one of them."

They discussed medication adjustments. Metformin reduced by 50%. Blood pressure medication reduced. Check back in 30 days to potentially reduce further.

Marcus walked out and sat in his car for ten minutes.

Two months ago: limping at his daughter's wedding, four medications, pre-diabetic, heading toward a heart attack like his father.

Today: reversing everything. Not managing. Reversing.

He called Jennifer. "The labs came back."

"And?"

"Dr. Patel says I'm reversing metabolic syndrome. He's reducing my medications."

He heard her crying on the other end.

"I'm so proud of you. And relieved. I was so scared, Marcus."

"I know. Me too. But we're okay now."

James's Backyard - Saturday Morning

James stood in his garden holding a fishing rod. Tyler was beside him, practicing casting.

"Like this, Grandpa?"

"Exactly. Now flick your wrist—there! Perfect cast."

They were practicing for tomorrow's fishing trip. The one they'd been doing every Saturday for the past month. The one James thought he'd never be physically able to do.

Susan watched from the porch, wiping her eyes.

Later, after Tyler left, James showed Susan his lab results.

Kidney function:

- Three months ago: eGFR 52, Creatinine 1.4
- Today: eGFR 58, Creatinine 1.2

"Your kidneys improved," Susan said, staring at the numbers.

"The doctor said kidney function at my stage doesn't improve. He called me himself. Wanted to know exactly what I was doing."

James looked at his hands. "Sue, my hands don't hurt. I built that birdhouse. I'm working in the garden for hours. I'm taking Tyler fishing every week and I'm not worried about whether I can do it. I know I can."

"How's your uric acid?"

"7.3. Not perfect, but down from 10.1. And I haven't had a flare in sixty-three days."

Susan hugged him. "You did it, Jim."

"We did it. You did this with me every step."

Your Complete 90-Day Comparison

Pull out everything from Day 1.

The Numbers

Weight and Measurements:

	Weight	Waist	Chest	Hips
Day 1				
Day 90				
Change				

Lab Results (if available):

Uric Acid: _____ → _____
eGFR: _____ → _____
Fasting Glucose: _____ → _____
A1C: _____ → _____
CRP: _____ → _____
Cholesterol: _____ → _____
Blood Pressure: _____ → _____

Pain Tracking:

Day 1 Average: _____/10
Day 90 Average: _____/10
Pain-free days Week 1: _____
Pain-free days Week 12: _____
Total flares in 90 days: _____

Energy & Sleep:

Day 1 Energy: _____/10 | Day 90: _____/10
Day 1 Sleep: _____ hours, _____/10 quality
Day 90 Sleep: _____ hours, _____/10 quality

Beyond the Numbers

Activities I couldn't do on Day 1 that I can do now:

1. ______________________________
2. ______________________________
3. ______________________________
4. ______________________________
5. ______________________________

How I feel different (not just physically):

___

What others have said:

___

My proudest moment:

___

The Photo Comparison

Look at your Day 1 photos. Compare to Day 90.

What do you notice?

- Face: Less puffy? Y / N
- Posture: Standing taller? Y / N
- Body: Visible changes? Y / N
- Energy: Look more vibrant? Y / N

The photos don't lie. Neither do the measurements. But the real transformation is how you FEEL when you look at them.

Lessons Learned

About Your Body

My biggest trigger foods: ___

Foods I thought were bad but are fine: ___

My optimal sleep amount: ___

How stress affects my pain: ___

About Yourself

What surprised me most: ______________________

What was easier than expected: ______________________

What was harder than expected: ______________________

My biggest strength: ______________________

How I've grown: ______________________

About Change

What I would tell Day 1 me: ______________________

What I would do differently: ______________________

What I would do the same: ______________________

The most important lesson: ______________________

Your Success Story

Write it down. For yourself. For others. For the future you who might forget how far you've come.

My 90-Day Transformation Story:

Where I started: ______________________

Why I committed: ______________________

The hardest moments: ______________________

The breakthrough moments: ______________________

Where I am now: ______________________________

What this means for my future: ______________________________

The Ripple Effect

Your transformation doesn't just affect you.

Who have you influenced?

- Family members who notice: ______________________
- Friends who asked questions: ______________________
- Coworkers who want to learn: ______________________
- Others you've inspired: ______________________

Elena started a walking group that grew to 12 people.
Marcus's wife transformed alongside him.
James helped 5 church members start their journeys.

Your transformation creates permission for others to change.

What Happens Now

Day 90 isn't the end. It's the beginning of your new normal.

Your Next 90 Days (Days 91-180)
Goals:
Maintain:

- ____
- ____

Improve:

- ______________________________

Explore:

- ______________________________

Share:

- ______________________________

Your One-Year Vision

By Day 365, I will:

Health-wise: ______________________________

Physically capable of: ______________________________

Living this way: ______________________________

Helping others by: ______________________________

Your Life Vision

Five years from now:

My health will allow me to: ______________________________

I'll be grateful I started because: ______________________________

The life I'm living will include: ______________________________

Final Words

Ninety days ago, you made a decision. Not just to manage gout. To reclaim your life.

Some of you started skeptical. Some desperate. Some hopeful but uncertain. All of you committed.

You learned that your body isn't the enemy. It's not broken. It's not betraying you. It's just responding to how you treat it.

You learned that change doesn't require perfection. It requires consistency. Small actions, repeated daily, compound into transformation.

You learned that the hard part isn't knowing what to do. It's doing it anyway when it's difficult. When you're tired. When no one's watching. When results feel slow.

And you did it anyway.

You proved:

You're capable of more than you thought.
You're stronger than you believed.
Your body can heal when given what it needs.
Change is possible at any age, any condition, any circumstance.
Ninety days can change your life.

But more importantly, you learned:

This isn't about 90 days. It's about the rest of your life.
You're not "done." You're just beginning.
The protocol trained you. Now you live it.
Not perfectly. Not rigidly. Not obsessively.
Just healthily. Sustainably. Joyfully.
Welcome to the rest of your life.

You're not managing gout anymore.

You're living free.

TAKE ACTION: Your Day 90 Celebration

Document Everything

- Take Day 90 photos (same poses as Day 1)
- Record all measurements
- Complete comparison worksheet
- Write your success story
- Save all data for future reference

Celebrate Appropriately

Choose a celebration that honors your journey:

- Buy new clothes that fit your transformed body
- Book that activity you couldn't do on Day 1
- Plan a healthy celebration meal
- Share your story with someone who inspired you
- Do something physical that demonstrates your capability
- Write a letter to Day 1 you
- Start helping someone else begin

Elena's celebration: Signed up for another 5K with Sofia
Marcus's celebration: Weekend trip with Jennifer, hiking
James's celebration: Built that birdhouse with Tyler

Set Your Course Forward

- Review your maintenance plan
- Schedule your first quarterly check-in (Day 180)
- Commit to annual tune-up protocol
- Identify one person you might help
- Write your Day 365 goals

Share Your Story (If You Want)

Consider:

- Posting in online communities
- Telling your doctor (they need success stories)
- Inspiring family/friends
- Documenting for your future self

You don't have to. But your story might be exactly what someone else needs to hear.

One Last Thing

Three people started this journey with you, at least in these pages.

Elena, who couldn't walk without pain, who missed her daughter's life, who felt like her best years were behind her. Today she runs. She's present. She's alive.

Marcus, who was heading toward his father's fate, who chose work over health, who couldn't enjoy life because he was too sick. Today he's reversed metabolic syndrome. He works four days a week. He has decades ahead of him.

James, who thought 61 was too old to change, whose body was failing, who couldn't play with his grandson. Today his kidneys are improving. He fishes every weekend. He's building that birdhouse next Saturday.

Three different people. Three different stories. Three different lives.

All transformed in 90 days.

Your story is just as important.

Whether you lost 15 pounds or 30. Whether you're pain-free or just significantly better. Whether you're off medication or on less. Whether you ran a 5K or just walked around the block without limping.

You transformed.

And transformation, once begun, continues.

The question isn't "What did I accomplish in 90 days?"

The question is "What will I do with the rest of my healthy life?"

The answer is yours to write.

Day 90. Not the end. The beginning.

Welcome to your gout-free future.

You earned it.

"Day 90 is when I realized the protocol wasn't something I did. It was someone I became." — Elena Martinez

"The data proves the transformation. But the feeling of waking up pain-free proves that life is worth optimizing for." — Marcus Chen

"I thought I was too old. Turns out, I was just not trying. Now I'm living proof that it's never too late." — James Morrison

---

THE END

(Or, more accurately, THE BEGINNING)

APPENDIX:

QUICK REFERENCE GUIDES

Purine Content Food Chart

HIGH PURINE AVOID (>200mg per 100g)	MODERATE PURINE - CAUTION (100-200mg per 100g)	LOWER PURINE - GENERALLY SAFE (50-100mg per 100g)	LOW PURINE - SAFE (<50mg per 100g)
Organ meats (liver, kidney, brain, sweetbreads)	Beef, pork, lamb	Chicken, turkey	**Proteins** Eggs (all forms)
Anchovies	Duck, goose	Ham	All dairy (milk, cheese, yogurt)
Sardines (canned in oil)	Bacon	Salmon, cod, halibut	Tofu
Herring	Veal	Bass	**Vegetables (ALL SAFE)**
Mackerel (Atlantic)	Shellfish (lobster, crab, shrimp)		Asparagus, mushrooms, spinach (high purine but plant-based = safe)
Game meats (venison, rabbit, wild boar)	Tuna, trout, haddock		Peas, beans, lentils (protective despite purines)
Meat extracts and gravies	Scallops		**Fruits**: All safe
Yeast extracts			**Grains**: All safe
			Fats/Oil: All safe
			Nuts/Seeds: All safe

KEY INSIGHT: Plant purines ≠ Animal purines. Focus on food quality, not just purine content.

Anti-Inflammatory Foods Rating

SUPER (Eat Daily)	HIGH (Excellent Choices)	MODERATE	AVOID
Fatty fish (salmon, mackerel, sardines)	Other fish (cod, halibut)	Eggs	Refined sugar
Berries (blueberries, strawberries, blackberries)	Chicken (pasture-raised preferred)	Greek yogurt	Refined grains (white bread, white rice, white pasta)
Tart cherries	Cruciferous vegetables (broccoli, Brussels sprouts, cauliflower)	Other vegetables	Seed oils (vegetable, canola, soybean, corn)
Leafy greens (kale, spinach, chard)	Tomatoes (cooked)	Most fruits	Trans fats
Turmeric	Bell peppers	Whole grains (quinoa, oats)	Processed meats
Ginger (fresh)	Garlic, onions	Sweet potatoes	Fried foods
Extra virgin olive oil	Walnuts, almonds	Grass-fed beef (small amounts)	Fast food
Green tea	Chia seeds, flaxseeds		Excessive alcohol
Dark chocolate (70%+ cacao)	Beans and lentils		
Avocados	Coconut oil		
	Fresh herbs (rosemary, oregano, basil)		

Emergency Flare Protocol

IMMEDIATE (0-4 hours):

1. Stop current activity, rest joint
2. Elevate affected area if possible
3. Ice for 20 minutes (not directly on skin)
4. Drink 16 oz water immediately
5. Take prescribed flare medication if available
6. Do NOT take NSAIDs if you have kidney concerns

NEXT 24 HOURS:

1. Increase water to 120 oz
2. Cherry juice every 4 hours
3. Stick to safest foods only
4. Gentle movement (not affected joint)
5. Track what preceded flare
6. Rest more than usual
7. Avoid all alcohol
8. Reduce stress (cancel non-essentials)

DAYS 2-3:

1. Continue high hydration
2. Return to Phase 1 basics
3. Gentle stretching (not affected joint)
4. Review last 72 hours for triggers
5. Doctor visit if not improving

WHEN TO CALL DOCTOR:

- Fever with flare
- Flare lasting >5 days
- New joint affected

- Severe swelling/redness
- Can't bear any weight
- Symptoms worsening

Shopping Staples Master List

PROTEINS (Always Have)	VEGETABLES
☐ Chicken breast/thighs	☐ Mixed greens/spinach
☐ Ground turkey	☐ Broccoli, cauliflower
☐ Eggs	☐ Bell peppers
☐ Salmon (fresh or frozen)	☐ Onions, garlic
☐ Canned salmon/sardines	☐ Carrots, celery
☐ Rotisserie chicken (backup)	☐ Cucumber, tomatoes
	☐ Frozen mixed vegetables
FRUITS	**FATS**
☐ Berries (frozen in bulk)	☐ Extra virgin olive oil
☐ Apples, pears	☐ Avocado oil
☐ Lemons (always!)	☐ Coconut oil
☐ Avocados (various ripeness)	☐ Butter
☐ Bananas	☐ Nuts (almonds, walnuts)
	☐ Seeds (chia, flax)
	☐ Almond/nut butter
PANTRY	**SPICES (Build Over Time)**
☐ Quinoa, wild rice	☐ Sea salt, black pepper
☐ Oats (steel-cut or rolled)	☐ Turmeric, ginger
☐ Canned beans (black, kidney)	☐ Cinnamon, cumin
☐ Canned tomatoes	☐ Paprika, chili powder
☐ Coconut milk	☐ Garlic powder, onion powder
☐ Chicken/vegetable broth	☐ Oregano, basil, rosemary, thyme
☐ Apple cider vinegar	
☐ Coconut aminos	

HYDRATION

☐ Tart cherry juice

☐ Herbal teas

☐ Sparkling water

Final Quick Reference: The Essentials

IF YOU REMEMBER NOTHING ELSE:

✓ Eat real food, mostly plants, quality protein

✓ Drink 80-100 oz water daily

✓ Move 15-30 minutes daily

✓ Sleep 7-8 hours nightly

✓ Manage stress actively

✓ Track pain/energy to stay aware

✓ Avoid processed sugar, refined grains, seed oils

✓ Return to protocol immediately after any deviation

✓ Progress over perfection

✓ Your body can heal when you give it what it needs

Keep this page visible. Reference it daily until it's automatic.

A Note to Readers

Thank you so much for reading!

If you enjoyed this book found it to be helpful, I would be truly grateful if you could take a moment to leave an honest review on Amazon.

Your feedback not only helps other readers discover the book, but also supports the creation of more practical, accessible guides like this one.

Thank you for being part of the journey.

Made in the USA
Monee, IL
13 September 2026

62976630R00118